THE SEARCH FOR THE PERFECT PROTEIN

THE
SEARCH FOR THE PERFECT PROTEIN

THE KEY TO **SOLVING** WEIGHT LOSS, DEPRESSION, FATIGUE, INSOMNIA, AND OSTEOPOROSIS

Dr. David Minkoff

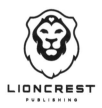

LIONCREST
PUBLISHING

THE SEARCH FOR THE PERFECT PROTEIN
*The Key to Solving Weight Loss, Depression,
Fatigue, Insomnia, and Osteoporosis*

ISBN   978-1-5445-0386-8 *Paperback*
   978-1-5445-0385-1 *Ebook*

This book is dedicated to all of the wonderful mentors who opened my eyes to biological medicine—the science of restoring life and livingness to our species and planet. Biology, as life, only exists where there is cooperation between cells and earth and sunlight and beings. Our modern medicine and culture have become anti-biology in many respects, and in their wake our species and planet are in great peril. It is my hope that we can turn this tide and bring ourselves, our medicine, and our cultures back to life so our future generations can enjoy this Garden of Eden that we have been blessed to inhabit.

To Sue, the love of my life of fifty years, and my partner in learning and fun. To my three amazing children Uri, Max, and Rebecca, and our eight grandchildren who support and inspire me every day, provide me with their unconditional love and support, and permit the future to be eternally bright.

CONTENTS

FOREWORD

I first met Dr. David Minkoff when I visited his office in Clearwater, Florida, and he gave me a fascinating tour of a true, cutting-edge, anti-aging facility. Since that time, I've gotten to know the good doctor on a much deeper level, and I realize that he is far ahead of his time in the areas of true enhancement and healing of the human body. He has extreme knowledge of essential amino acids and how they interact with nearly every aspect of physiology, so when I heard that he was writing a book on proteins and amino acids, I sat back and waited with bated breath.

As expected, Dr. Minkoff delivered. Upon reviewing the original manuscript for what you are about to read, I was blown away. Reading this book will completely reinvent the way you think about your body digesting and assimilating proteins. You'll discover the wonderful world of amino acids—particularly essential amino acids—and the little-known ways they can heal your gut, recover your muscle, enhance your neurotransmitters, and support healing from a wide variety of chronic diseases and issues.

After Dr. Minkoff taught me the facts about how amino acids trump popular alternative products such as protein powder and collagen, I have adopted a habit of consuming twenty to forty grams of amino acids per day, and I've witnessed a profound transformation in the realms of mental function, workout recovery, endurance and strength training performance, sleep, and gut stability. I was even able to compete in six Ironman triathlons, including three Ironman World Championships, using a purely ketogenic diet, forgoing sugary gels, goos, and energy bars. I relied upon amino acids as my primary secret weapon, instead. This type of protocol currently flies under the radar in the supplement industry, but I predict that over the next decade, the use of essential amino acids will take the world by storm. After reading this book, you will be equipped and empowered with every shred of knowledge you need to take full advantage of this little-known superfood. Dr. Minkoff has elegantly woven together everything you need to know, so sit back and enjoy the ride!

Ben Greenfield, MS, CSCS
CEO Kion
BenGreenfieldFitness.com

FOREWORD

I wanted to become an Olympian when I was seven years old. I thought it would be the coolest thing ever to march in the opening day ceremony parade, walk into the Olympic stadium, and see the lighting of the torch.

With the help of family, friends, mentors and benefactors, I fulfilled my dream of becoming an Olympian. I represented the USA overseas in the Munich, Germany Olympics as a cyclist. I marched into the Olympic stadium during the opening day ceremony.

After the Olympics, I went on to complete my master's degree in sports science at the University of Southern California and became a sports chiropractor. Then, I started my professional career as an advisor to athletes— the ones who become Olympic champions, highly paid professionals, help teams win world championships, and guide businesspeople to become business icons. My clients went on to win over forty Olympic, world, national, and Tour de France championships.

At that point, I thought I was doing well. Olympics: check. Master's in Sports Science and a successful career: check. Identify need, get more education, fill void: check. I'd met and exceeded all my major goals and expectations for my life, but then, something happened.

At the height of my career, I developed a rash on my arms and legs that randomly came and went. The medical experts I consulted offered me a variety of diagnoses, ranging from adrenal fatigue to systemic mold infection. None of their treatments helped, and my health began to deteriorate rapidly over the next couple of years until I was incapacitated. I couldn't function mentally or physically, and I was at the lowest point in my life.

Then, I met David Minkoff, MD, and everything changed.

David's credentials were impeccable: he was a medical doctor with advanced training in pediatrics, had been an emergency room doc, and was on the leading edge of environmental medicine. He had a track record of restoring health to those who weren't finding healing through mainstream medical care.

After telling David about my health challenges, he invited me to come and stay at with him and his family at his home in Clearwater, Florida, and he'd evaluate me at his clinic, Lifeworks Wellness Center. He concluded that I had mercury poisoning from my silver-mercury dental fillings, came up with a healing protocol, and assured me that I would get well.

His treatment worked.

David's protocol healed me, but that's not all that happened. I learned more about health and performance while under his care than I had in thousands of hours spent in school!

His care showed me that the body can heal itself when all of its systems work together as a holistic, single, super-system. The healing program included IVs, personalized diets, supplements, allergy desensitization, ozone therapy, neural therapy, and electromagnetic modalities to restore my body. These methods were so effective that I used several of them when I cared for the Tour de France teams and supported racer recovery after each of its brutal twenty-one days.

We won eight straight Tours.

Because of the results I experienced personally and witnessed with the Tour teams, I began referring patients to

David. I can honestly say that David's track record borders on the unbelievable. He cured patients who had suffered years of pain and frustration. He gave hope to people that most traditional doctors considered hopeless. More importantly, he gave them their health which is priceless.

His results are no accident: David is a dedicated student of his chosen discipline. He continuously attends post-graduate conferences and seminars on topics he deems interesting or potentially helpful. He's a voracious reader and devours all the latest clinical publications. He dedicates all his spare time to discovering how to make extraordinary clinical outcomes the norm. I tell everyone that he's the smartest person I know. My wife refers to him as a "living treasure" because of his knowledge, genius, and dedication to the art of healing.

David also practices what he preaches; he's competed in more triathlons than I can count over the past several decades. To sum it all up, David is a renaissance man and a leader in his industry.

My advice? Whatever David is doing, take notice. Decades of success prove you can't go wrong!

Dr. Jeff Spencer, M.A., D.C.
Creator of the Goal Achievement Roadmap™ and Champion's Mindset™

FOREWORD

I have known and worked closely with Dr. David Minkoff for well over two decades. We have worked together to help some of the sickest patients, suffering from some of the worst possible diseases, including cancer. Dr. Minkoff has been tireless in his pursuit to find the true causes of disease, and what to do about it in the safest and most natural way possible. He and I have been doing this for a long time; I admire his tenacity, and I like the way he thinks!

After reading the manuscript for the first time, I was thankful to Dr. Minkoff for putting these materials together so succinctly and understandably. In this book, he takes the cloak of mystery off the subject of proteins, making a potentially complicated subject much easier to understand. It is an excellent synopsis of the most important fundamentals about essential amino acids that every nutrition-oriented health care provider needs to know. It is written in a style that is both friendly and inviting—it practically reads like a good novel that you don't want to put down until the end. How unusual for a book on such a technical matter!

I have trained thousands of doctors in the field of nutrition and functional medicine for over twenty-five years, and my work and training programs continue to grow each year; I am looking forward to including this book in our training materials. I know it will be enjoyed and valuable to every dedicated nutrition-oriented health care provider. Dr. Minkoff's extensive knowledge and expertise in the field of essential amino acids and their impact on vital body functions, from detox to repair and regeneration, translates to increased understanding of this important subject on a patient-by-patient basis.

We want to evolve from the current symptom suppression/ disease maintenance model to a truly effective, workable method to restore health and help each patient maintain it through the most natural means possible. This is a goal I am sure we can all agree upon, and one which we are mutually dedicated to bringing into existence. This book contributes to that forward motion by simplifying and clarifying that which can help improve the lives of our patients even more.

Freddie Ulan, DC, CCN
Founder of Ulan Nutritional Systems & Nutrition Response Testing®

FOREWORD

I just finished a sixty-mile bike ride, followed by a three-mile run on a tough, hilly course. It was four and a half hours of hard, non-stop work. I'm a triathlete who races, so this is just one of my normal workouts—nothing special. Except for one little thing: I'm seventy-four years old.

I consider this as just part of a day in my active life, but I'm not naive enough to think this is the norm for folks my age. Old classmates and friends I've grown up with remind me every day of what many people this age contend with: lack of mobility, reduced activity, constant aches and pains, and the list goes on and on.

Fortunately, I'm too busy to spend much time asking why I'm still enjoying a physically active life while others are not so lucky. But I do have a few thoughts on the subject.

Of course, it all begins with some good genes, for which I can take absolutely no credit, but will thank Mom and Dad. And my folks did take it one step further. Dinner in my home, unlike in Dr. Minkoff's, was not a place where food was the focal point. Rather, it was a time to fill your belly and get going again. It wasn't necessarily healthy food (hot dogs were a staple) but it wasn't slathered with gravy, nor was there too much of it. And the only desserts I ate as a kid were the ones I could score at a friend's house. Make no mistake about it, there was not much thought being given to good health—other than having to drink milk at every meal—but it was keeping me lean and, somehow, teaching me something about healthy eating (not counting the hot dogs)!

Being active was considered the only acceptable behavior in my household. Reading was good, but only after the sun went down. If there was a hint of daylight, we kids were expected to be outside playing. I may be exaggerating a bit here because doing well in school was also key, but you get the picture. I learned that an active lifestyle was the norm.

During my twenties, thirties, and forties, I focused on my career, and in my mid-forties, I started marathon running. Looking back, I believe it was a natural evolution after all of that running around as a kid. But I did make an interesting discovery when I started running: I found that I had some athletic chops. A few years later, the running led to IRONMAN racing, a sport about which I was passionate. And that's where I met Dr. Minkoff, a forty-two-time Ironman finisher.

In 2002, I was struggling with a balky hamstring. I had tried all of the usual remedies, but just couldn't get it under control; I was willing to try anything. I read an article by Dr. Minkoff about using an amino acid product to help this kind of injury, and it made sense to me, so I tried it, hoping it would be a lifeline. It wasn't long before the hamstring was no longer an issue, and I also noticed that I was having very good back-to-back-to-back workouts. It seemed that my recovery between hard bouts was happening faster than it did previously. That was the beginning of my "love affair" with *Perfect Amino*. I've been using it religiously since then, and I strongly believe it is a huge contributor to my being able to keep a consistent, challenging training schedule as I've aged.

Dr. Minkoff is a familiar figure as a medical practitioner and in the endurance world. Now, he's taken his unique experiences in both fields and written a book on living energetically. He speaks passionately about how each of us can learn more about our bodies, and how to pursue good health to support an active lifestyle. He takes a complex subject and makes it very understandable to the layman who is interested in living well today and tomorrow. Whether you're a seventy-four-year-old tri-athlete or a young, hard-working professional, it's a very encouraging view of life!

Cherie Gruenfeld
IRONMAN World Champion
Author of *Become an Ironman*

FOREWORD

Whoever said, "There's no such thing as a free lunch," was right on the money. According to what I could find, the term was first used by an economist by the name of Harley L. Lutz. Mr. Lutz was referring to the fact that nothing good comes without a price. Somewhere, somehow, somebody has got to pay. Now, while that concept is certainly true of economics, it is also true for health. If you want to be healthy, you are going to have to pay for it. Sorry, but it's true—there really is no free lunch! So, what kind of payments are we talking about?

First of all, there is sacrifice. If you smoke, you will have to stop. If you like eating nutrient poor, processed, GMO foods, you will have to stop. If you like to stay up and watch TV instead of going to sleep, you will have to stop. If you like to drink beer instead of water, you will have to change that too. I could go on and on, but you get the point. If you want to be healthy, somebody is going to have to pay the bill. And that somebody can only be you.

Next, you have to spend money. Oh, no! Oh, yes. Good food costs more. Exercise equipment is not free. Supplements cost money. Health books and newsletters are not free either. Preventive medical visits and lab tests are not usually covered by insurance; for the most part, they are an extra expense. The question is, are you willing to part with some bucks in order to stay healthy and free of disease? I will never forget a patient I saw thirty-five years ago, when I was just a neophyte in the world of preventive medicine. I told her she needed to start taking a few supplements every day. She asked me what it would cost, and I told her fifty-five dollars. She said, "Isn't there something else I can do? That seems like too much." And then later in the visit, she told me that she couldn't make her next appointment because she and her husband would be on a four-week cruise!

Lastly, there is work. Being healthy requires some work. Most people don't want to work for free. They want to get paid for their time. I'll bet that if the government paid everyone fifty dollars for every mile they ran, the "healthcare crisis" would mysteriously go away. About three years ago, I was at my local gym, stressing and straining. I wasn't working for free though. I was getting paid big time. That sweat pays good dividends in terms of preventing disease and staying strong. Over in the bike section, there were two senior citizens riding stationary bikes side by side. They were both sipping on a cup of coffee while gabbing and turning the cranks at the slowest speed possible. They were at the gym, but they were not working, and as a result they were not getting paid. That's a bad deal.

There is no free lunch. That's the bad news. But the good news is this: things are changing.

I've been practicing medicine for almost fifty years now, and things are different today. In the past, a good day at the office was when the waiting room was filled with sick people. Now, a good day at the office is when my patients are coming in not because of a health problem, but instead are coming in while they are healthy to learn how to stay that way. These people know all too well about the "free lunch" thing. And they are more than willing to pay for a fully functional, energetic life that is free of disease. Unlike the patient who could afford a four-week cruise but couldn't afford fifty dollars per month for supplements, I had a patient come in last week who said, "Doc, I don't care what it costs, and I don't care what I have to do. I want to live long and strong." That is the "patient" of the future. If you have that kind of attitude, then Dr. Minkoff has done you a good service. That's because he has captured the missing link that virtually no one has talked about: the perfect protein.

As far as I know, this is the first book written for a general audience that focuses on protein. When I first heard Dr. Minkoff lecture on the concepts in this book almost six years ago, I was completely amazed. At that time, I had been practicing alternative, nutritional medicine for thirty some odd years, and I had never heard this information before. All proteins are not the same. For one, many protein sources end up being wasted because they are not digested effectively. And then there is the issue of the amino acid balance in different protein sources. If the balance is not right, up to 70 percent of the protein can be wasted. For these reasons and others, many people are protein deficient and don't even know it.

Dr. Minkoff correctly points out that virtually everyone who has a chronic ailment is protein deficient. That can come about either as the cause or effect of the illness, but in either event, it needs to be fixed so the person can get well. For many patients, the difference between getting well and staying strong and healthy versus inviting disease has to do with eating the right protein. Protein deficiency leads to fatigue, weakness, tissue breakdown, hair loss, muscle wasting, gastrointestinal complaints, mental symptoms such as depression, anxiety, decreased cognitive function, insomnia, decreased balance, bone loss, rapid aging, environmental sensitivity, Parkinson's, dementia, premature aging, and disease. And while you think you may be getting enough of the right protein, odds are that you are not.

Another thing that is great about *The Search for the Perfect Protein* is that it is unusual to read a book that has specific information for all kinds of people including those who are sick, pregnant women, children, old folks, athletes, and young people. Getting the right amount and right kind of protein is critical for us all. You can have everything else right, but if you get protein wrong, you will have problems.

So, read these pages with great enthusiasm. The stories are telling, the science is there, and the solution is surprising. One of the original pioneers in nutritional medicine was Adelle Davis. Look her up. One of her sayings was "As I see it, every day you do one of two things: build health or produce disease in yourself." I think of that often. And, while our entire medical system is focused on treating disease instead of preventing it, I'll leave you with one of my own sayings: "The best treatment for any disease is not to get it." Getting the right protein in your body is one of the best ways to accomplish that. If there is a free lunch, then that's it!

Frank Shallenberger, MD

Author of *Bursting with Energy* and *The Type 2 Diabetes Breakthrough*

Editor of *Second Opinion* Newsletter

President of American Academy of Ozonotherapy

NOTE FROM THE AUTHOR

Dear Reader,

I was stuck. I was searching...

I had fourteen years of post-high school medical education, but didn't have the answers. I sought advice from countless practitioners. They didn't have the answers, either.

I knew what didn't work. But I didn't know what *would* work. I was in search of the perfect protein that would heal my body and take me to the next level.

Have you ever been in such a situation? Where you knew there had to be an answer, but it kept eluding you? What did you do? You searched and searched, and you searched some more.

Herein is my search, and what I found. It has helped me, and beyond that, tens of thousands of others.

If you have been searching, God willing, it will help you too.

Good luck,

DM

INTRODUCTION

THE ANSWER I STUMBLED UPON

Like most children, I learned about nutrition from my parents and extended family. The education was daily, from meal to meal as practical instruction. My parents learned what "good food" was from their parents, and they liked whatever tasted good. It was that simple.

I was brought up in a Midwestern, Jewish home, where all of the most important activities revolved around meal time and food. It didn't matter if the occasion was happy or sad, serious or playful; everyone ate as if it were their last meal, and until their stomachs bulged. Even though their bellies were full, the thought of when and where the next meal would occur was on everyone's mind. Food was a complement to all events, and the antidote to life's problems.

My Russian-immigrant grandparents served an abundance of traditional heavy foods including fatty meats, starches saturated with drippings or chicken fat, and sugary desserts. Salads and vegetables were nowhere to be found on their table, with the exception of potatoes, creamed and buttered to their delight. We had a kosher home where the dietary laws prohibited milk and meat in the same meal, but my mother insisted we drink milk with every meal—we needed calcium so "our bones would grow strong." I don't know if she believed this because we lived in Wisconsin, the Dairy State, or because our milkman was an exceptional salesman. Milk always gave me a stomachache, but my complaints were ignored, so I learned to live with it. Those were the days when children "should be seen and not heard," and our opinions were certainly never asked for or acknowledged. "Clean your plate! There are many children in China who are going hungry," was another of the familiar maxims.

As a good boy, I complied until I was fourteen. My Boy Scout troop visited the Oscar Meyer headquarters in my hometown of Madison, Wisconsin, and it was an eye-opening experience. We never ate pork, and merely uttering the word in our house created a feeling of disgust, but the sight of pigs being hit one-by-one over the head with large mallets and then slaughtered sickened me. That was the day I decided to become a vegetarian.

As you can imagine, this did not go over well with my mother. She took it as a personal affront that I would no longer eat her cooking. When I wouldn't let up on my decision, she put me through a number of trials to get me to change my mind. She even revoked my car privileges for a year because I wouldn't eat what the family ate! She worried that my health would suffer due to my lack of protein—she dragged me to the doctor for blood tests every few months to check for anemia and other nutritional deficiencies. It was no matter that nearly all of my relatives had heart attacks at relatively young ages; the nutritional truths and dictums of the family could not be challenged. And certainly not by a questioning teenager.

Even though nobody at home supported my lifestyle, I stuck with my decision. I met my future wife, Sue, around this time, and I went to her house frequently for meals. Her family was from Alsace, an area between the French and German border, and their food traditions were completely different from that of my family's. They loved making things that I liked to eat, and didn't care for forcing meat down my throat. Alice, my future mother-in-law, came from generations of bakers, and she made fresh and hot breads or croissants daily. They also served wonderful fresh salad greens, asparagus, and green beans from their backyard garden.

Her dad, Leo, was a cattle dealer, and he brought home

fresh, non-pasteurized milk several times a week. Alice made her own cottage cheese and butter, and desserts were fresh baked pies made with homegrown berries and rhubarb. I ate with them as often as I could. Their support and the variety of foods they offered only increased my love for vegetables, and I continued my life as a vegetarian.

THE LINK BETWEEN FOOD AND HEALTH

For thousands of years, cultures never disputed whether certain foods were healthy or not. For much of history, people were just happy to have a meal. Geographic areas, ethnic traditions, and the need for pure survival over the centuries proved the acceptable diet; the various peoples of earth had their own nourishing traditions. This was often due to necessity—each culture had its staples, and they ate them because they were available. In the early 1900s, heart disease, cancer, autism and autoimmune diseases were rare occurrences. Conditions like osteoporosis and diabetes were practically unheard of. Only in recent history has the relationship between food and health been recognized. Perhaps this is because the tried and true dietary habits of people have changed so drastically. Once upon a time, food was grown from a fertile earth without chemicals or genetically modified seeds and eaten locally and seasonally. Now, that has all changed.

Corporate industry has invaded the production of food and changed the pattern that had existed over millions of years. Now, family farms are rare and organic home gardens are even more so. Over the last seventy-five years, pseudoscientists have conducted paid "studies" that have been skewed to fit academic or corporate agendas for the purpose of making money—they hardly have any regard for health or environmental consequences. Most are inherently flawed, and designed to influence our food choices based on false findings. The results are bought and paid for before the experiments are even done! Such studies have led to popular, incorrect theories.

For example, you've probably heard that GMO Canola oil is good, saturated fats like butter and egg yolks are bad, low-fat foods are good, and cholesterol is bad. Why use compost and cow manure for fertilizer when you can just add chemicals to the soil? And marigolds to keep pests away? Fooey on that, just spray some *Roundup*—it works better. These practices have led to unhealthy habits, and in my opinion, have caused the current epidemics of obesity, diabetes, cancer, autism, autoimmune disease, and heart disease.

I am not against progress, but someone has to examine the downstream effects of what is taking place. There are now an estimated eighty-thousand synthetic chemicals permeating our environment that have never been tested for safety in humans. We breathe them, eat them as additives in our food, and put them on our hair and skin. Fathom for a moment that 2.6 billion pounds of glyphosate (Roundup) has been sprayed on U.S. farms in the past two decades.[1] Not only is this a risk to unsuspecting humans, it is killing off the soil's natural biome which is the source of all life on this planet.

1   Bellon, Tina, "Monsanto ordered to pay $289 million in world's first Roundup cancer trial," Reuters.com, August 8, 2018, https://www.reuters.com/article/us-monsanto-cancer-lawsuit/monsanto-ordered-to-pay-289-million-in-worlds-first-roundup-cancer-trial-idUSKBN1KV2HB

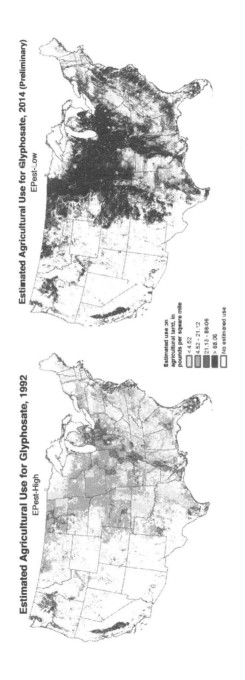

Estimated Agricultural Use for Glyphosate, 2014 (Preliminary)
EPest-Low

Estimated Agricultural Use for Glyphosate, 1992
EPest-High

Estimated use on
agricultural land, in
pounds per square mile
< 4.52
4.52 - 21.12
21.13 - 88.06
> 88.06
No estimated use

When we test the levels of glyphosate in the urine of average urban patients, we often find results like the following:

Glyphosate Profile

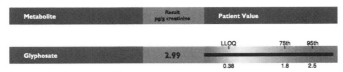

Metabolite	Result pg/g creatinine	Patient Value
Glyphosate	2.99	LLOQ 0.38 75th 1.8 95th 2.5

Should the food we eat and the environment we live in be so toxic that ordinary citizens have toxic amounts of chemicals in their bodies?

In fact, glyphosate is so harmful that Monsanto, the agrochemical company that developed *Roundup*, once had to pay a $39 million settlement to a gardener named Duane Johnson, a forty-six-year-old father of two. Johnson used the pesticide twenty to thirty times per year and was diagnosed with malignant lymphoma. The case against the company was that they had covered up the fact that *Roundup* was a carcinogen. Monsanto protested that eight-hundred studies had proven that the product was safe, but the jury saw through this charade of "bought and paid for science." The World Health Organization announced that Roundup was indeed probably carcinogenic to humans, and Johnson was awarded the settlement.[2]

---

2 Bellon, Tina, "Monsanto ordered to pay $289 million in world's first Roundup cancer trial," Reuters.com, August 8, 2018, https://www.reuters.com/article/us-monsanto-cancer-lawsuit/monsanto-ordered-to-pay-289-million-in-worlds-first-roundup-cancer-trial-idUSKBN1KV2HB

Fortunately, a detrimental disease isn't what led me to question and research the foods I was eating. After years of training for Ironman Triathlons, I sustained a hamstring injury that wouldn't heal. I was still a vegetarian at this time, and as a medical doctor, I did all I could to help it heal. I got massages, injections, chiropractic care, and went to physical therapy. I had access to every possible treatment, yet nothing worked. This led me to believe that maybe my mother was right (oh no!), and my vegetarian nutrition was hindering the healing process.

ANOTHER ENIGMA

During my search, a patient of mine, Pamela, an expert in cancer nutrition, told me of a protocol that could detect if a person was in the early stages of cancer—it consisted of taking concentrated pancreatic enzymes for three days. According to the theory, cancerous cells coat themselves with a protein so that the body's immune system doesn't recognize them as hostile; therefore, they are protected from being discovered and attacked. When taken, the concentrated pancreatic enzymes enter the bloodstream and are absorbed. The cancer's protein coat is then "digested off," exposing the harmful cells so they can be killed by the immune system.

One day, Pamela and I were discussing this treatment; she told me that if someone had subclinical cancer and did a three-day-trial with these enzymes, they would have symptoms. If this happened, they should continue taking the enzymes until they were well, and the cancer, so to speak, would be "nipped in the bud." It sounded interesting to me, so I decided to try it.

On the first day of the test, I took a dozen enzyme tablets on an empty stomach. Within fifteen minutes I felt as if my stomach was on fire. I honestly thought the enzymes had burned a hole in it! In my distress, I called Pamela and told her I would not be finishing the trial and was drinking aloe juice to keep the fire under control. I was supposed to take a dozen tablets six times a day for three days, and there was no way I was doing it—I was down for the count.

Now I had two conditions: an injured hamstring and a burned-up stomach, and I wasn't any closer to getting better. I couldn't explain to myself what had happened, so I filed it away as a reaction that my body had to something it didn't like or couldn't handle.

A BREAKTHROUGH

Sometime later, I ran into a friend of mine who had discovered a blend of amino acid tablets while he was in Europe. They were only sold in pharmacies and were made of pure pharmaceutical-grade ingredients. He said athletes took them and they were excited about their much-reduced healing times and improved strength. Then, he gave me a couple of bottles to try. I am an avid self-experimenter, so I went with it. I had competed in the Ironman World Championships eight times, and my annual goal was to return to the race. I needed fast enough times to qualify, and I'd never get there that year if I didn't get myself healed.

I started taking ten of the essential amino acid tablets twice per day, as my friend had instructed. I could tell within a few days that my body liked them. Week by week, I felt stronger and my hamstring pain was going away. After about six weeks, I decided to go to the track and give my leg a real test. Six hard quarter mile repeats later, I walked to my car elated. There was no pain and my legs had their spring back! The optimum protein nutrition of this unique blend of essential amino acids had healed me. I remember thinking, "I believe I've found the solution."

In the weeks that followed, I noticed other positive physical changes. My heart rate on a maximum heart rate challenge increased by twelve beats—it went from a stable 174 to 186 without any change in my training methods. It was due to the nutrition. And even though there was no visible difference in my body's appearance, I had gained ten pounds of lean body mass. I could not conceive of how this was possible, so I called the product formulator to discuss the changes I had experienced. He said that after years of inadequate nutrition as a vegetarian, the essential amino acids were filling in lean body mass deficiencies. My bones, liver, and heart now weighed more, and this was why I didn't look any different—my organs and tissues had simply increased in weight.

Five months after beginning the amino acids, I achieved a personal best at Ironman Canada in Penticton B.C. In my new and improved physical state, I began to wonder if my vegetarian, protein-deficient diet was the reason why the anti-cancer enzymes scorched my stomach. Could it be that the mucous lining in my stomach was inadequate, and that had also held back the healing of my hamstring? I very badly wanted to find out, so I decided to try the enzymes again. I followed the full protocol, twelve tablets, six times per day for three consecutive days. I had no adverse reactions, and my stomach was fine. I learned that because my overall body protein levels had normalized, the mucous layer in my stomach was better able to handle the enzymes. What a revelation! I thought, could this also be a key problem with my patients and their various conditions?

TESTING PATIENTS

Armed with my newfound knowledge and faith in these tablets, I started testing the amino acid levels of patients at my alternative medicine clinic, Lifeworks Wellness Center. Blood test results showed that almost everyone had inadequate levels of at least one of the eight essential amino acids—the ones that are critical for making protein in the body. The way the body protein mechanism works is that if even just one of the essential amino acids is not present in a food, or if it is in low levels in any food, the body will not utilize that food to make body protein very well. The unique feature of the amino acid blend I took was that each of the essential eight amino acids was represented in a very specific ratio, and it allowed the body to make any of its proteins in the amount that was needed. (We'll discuss more about this later).

I began giving patients these amino acids, and they had amazing, beneficial effects. Women reported that their hair was growing at a rapid rate, and they had to visit the beauty salon more frequently. Their nails grew at a much faster rate and were no longer brittle. Many people reported a great increase in energy. Athletes reported healing of chronic injuries (like me), a decrease in chronic pain, and performance improvement. Some patients who took the amino acids were vegetarian, others were not, but *all* were healing and experiencing incredible results. These findings were too good to be kept a secret; I had to share them with other athletes and medical professionals. I wrote an article for *Triathlete* magazine about my experiences with this perfect amino acid blend, and the response was overwhelming. Thousands of readers inquired about it and wanted to know how they could get some.

Shortly after that, I received an invitation to speak at the American College of Nutrition. I was excited, but my mentor strongly suggested I decline. He said the organization was strongly tied to the whey protein industry, and they would not like what I had to say about how poorly utilized whey protein was in comparison to the amino acid blend. Here's why he was concerned: When milk is made into cheese, it's divided into two proteins, casein (which is used to make the cheese) and whey (a liquid). Whey was considered to be a waste product for many years, until someone discovered its protein content. In order to give scientific credibility to whey, its producers sponsored scientists to show its validity as a protein supplement. It is true that it's well digested and well absorbed, but the body's ability to make human protein out of cow or goat whey protein is very limited. This is generally not known, but seeing as Madison Avenue is very persuasive, it is now a billion-dollar industry.

The American College of Nutrition is a professional organization consisting of medical doctors, Registered Dieticians, and PhDs in nutrition. They were interested in the information I shared during my talk and felt they could apply it to their clinical practices. They were fascinated to learn that whey was a low-quality protein (based on actual amino acid utilization) and that the essential amino acid formulation was the highest quality ever developed for utilization and protein synthesis. They couldn't believe they had never heard anything like this before. To most of these highly educated professionals, it was quite a revelation.

NOT ALL PROTEINS ARE CREATED EQUAL

I work with world-class athletes at my alternative medicine clinic and treat people who have cancer, auto-immune diseases, dementia, Parkinson's, Lyme Disease, and chronic fatigue. Interestingly, I've found that most of them, both the very well and the very sick, have either clinical or subclinical protein deficiencies. Many people don't suspect that they are deficient because symptoms can be subtle, such as poor nail quality, or lack of muscle development in response to exercise. Most show improvement once we increase their protein intake, correct their digestive enzymes, and address other deficiencies. A world-class athlete might experience a second-or-two improvement in race time; and a chronically ill person might have improved anemia, a boost in energy, or their body becomes able to detoxify.

If you haven't been feeling well for some time, or you feel you aren't functioning at a high physical or mental level, it means what you are eating isn't providing the nutrients you need to produce cellular energy for growth, repair and detoxification. Many people believe a specialty diet is the solution. Like me, they decide to become a vegetarian, or they try the Atkins, Keto, or Bulletproof diet. None of these diets are bad, but they don't solve what I call "the protein problem," which is twofold.

The first part of the problem is that most of our chicken, beef, lamb, and dairy products aren't from quality sources. We don't have great access to nontoxic proteins that won't harm us. So, the problem isn't just the foods we eat—it's also what *our food* eats! Cows are often fed genetically modified corn that's been sprayed with glyphosate. The same cows are given antibiotics and hormones and those substances become part of our food. There are better sources of protein available now, but I bet 98 percent of the population won't attempt to find them. Mass-produced, genetically modified food may taste good, but it's poison.

The second part of the problem is the widespread myth that all proteins are created equal. Twenty-eight grams of protein from tuna is *not* the same as twenty-eight grams from Greek yogurt—they do not have an equivalent amount of nutrition. By "nutrition," I mean quantities of essential amino acids that the body can turn into protein. The body can't convert the cow dairy protein into human protein as efficiently as it can with the tuna. We must be informed and choose our protein sources wisely, because we need a certain amount of this nutrient each day to function at a high level.

If you were to ask a dietician about the difference between sources of proteins, they'd probably tell you there isn't any. It's not even on their radar. For example, dieticians will tell a patient they need fifty-six grams of protein per day, and they can get it from whole wheat bread, peanut butter, a couple of eggs, and a tuna fish salad. It's true that they can get fifty-six grams protein from these sources, but they are not getting the correct amounts of essential amino acids for their body to build and maintain its protein structure. The real key is getting the correct ratio of grams of essential amino acids, so that the body can use them to build its own proteins. I'll fully explain this in the chapters to come.

THE GOAL OF THIS BOOK

Despite the various qualities and types of protein available, for many it doesn't actually add up to getting the body enough protein to function optimally. We've briefly discussed two reasons for this problem already: scarcity of clean protein and the body's need to digest and absorb it for full nutritional benefit. We'll discuss these in further detail in Part One of this book: The Protein Problem.

In Part Two, Specifying Problems for Subgroups, I'll share personal stories and case studies to illustrate how a lack of protein affects various populations. I'll discuss the many health issues I've encountered with patients and how essential amino acid supplementation brought healing and change to their bodies. Since I am the founder of BodyHealth, a wellness nutrition company, I will refer to a product called "Perfect Amino" throughout the book—it's the amino acid formulation I use personally and the one I used with the patients who are in the presented case studies.

Marketing for the protein industry is so prevalent and strong that no one ever questions it. My hope is that this book will debunk common myths and educate you about protein. I can almost guarantee that when you finish reading this book, you will know more than your doctor, dietician, or nutritionist about protein needs for a healthy or healing body. They don't teach this in universities, and if it wasn't for pure luck I never would have learned it either. I want you to begin making informed decisions about what to put into your body, so you can improve your health, enhance athletic performance, and meet your goals!

PART ONE

THE PROTEIN PROBLEM

CHAPTER ONE

WHAT PROTEINS ARE AND WHAT THEY DO

The Holy Bible is a spiritual treatise on the creation of the earth, life, and man. If I were to write a takeoff on that in terms of human biochemistry, it would be *"In the beginning was the word, and the word was 'amino.'"*

I don't intend for the above quote to be sacrilegious—I'm referring to "the beginning" in a biological sense. Whether you are an evolutionist or creationist, the truth is, amino acids *were* the beginning, as they are the building blocks of life. Whether by accident or through creation, somehow, they were formed. Amino acids were then assembled into the first proteins that were most likely *enzymes*. Enzymes facilitate chemical reactions to occur faster and specifically, and once they came into existence, they allowed for the manufacture of proteins; which allowed for the creation of more complex cells and organisms—essentially, the human body. In fact, the word protein is derived from the Greek word *proteus*, which means "primary."

Our bodies are incredibly complicated organisms made up of more than 100 trillion cells and at least fifty thousand different proteins. The average cell is a very complex, independent living thing with an internal chemical reaction rate of about two thousand times per second. Think about that for a minute! If you hired a computer wizard and asked him to design a program like the human body, it would have to coordinate 100,000,000,000,000 (trillion) cells with reaction rates at two thousand times per second, where every cell had to be in sync with every other one—each would have to be aware of what the other was doing at every moment. It would also have to be completely adaptable to cold and heat, whether on top of a mountain or at the bottom of the ocean. It would need to function while awake, asleep, running, wounded, or sitting still. It would have to control hormones, salt balance, cellular energy production, growth, repair, and on and on. There is no computer or computer maven that could possibly design this! If you think that molecules could achieve this by a series of accidents over the millennia, think again. This system is a result of the miracle of creation and life. The level of activity and coordination in the human body is impossible for us to comprehend!

DAILY STRESSORS OF LIFE

Our bodies undergo wear and tear on a daily basis due to chemical and traumatic stress—these attack and cause damage to the protein structure. Each cell must constantly repair proteins and other vital components to maintain its integrity. For example, during triathlon season, I train for my next event. I'll run for eighty minutes in ninety-degree heat, and then swim in the ocean for forty-five. Those environments and stressors are hostile to individual cells. The body has to deal with heat, sweating, energy production, salt balance, and hormonal support. That effort also causes a great deal of structural trauma and micro-tearing of my muscles and ligaments. If someone is protein malnourished, they could never handle that stress. They could overheat, feel dizzy, not sweat enough to cool their body, cramp, or get weak and faint. They might have GI stress with nausea, vomiting, or diarrhea, or even suffer a heart attack. Their muscles and ligaments might be sore for days, or they will deal with exhaustion.

These consequences don't just pertain to athletes. Other stressors coming from a boss, work deadlines, or an antagonistic spouse or children can cause similar cellular trauma. Medications of every variety are also huge sources of chemical stress in the body, because all medicines are toxins and cause cellular injury. If people work in an environment with pollutants, chemicals, pesticides, and eat and drink them, that is also part of the equation. There is no escaping any of this in our current life, and in order to live—and for sure to thrive—the body must deal with what is thrown at it, and at the heart of that is protein metabolism.

PROTEIN MALNOURISHMENT

My definition of protein malnourishment is having inadequate levels of serum essential amino acids to accomplish normalization of the body's protein requirements. A former patient of mine was very protein malnourished, and if she so much as lifted a book from a table, her arm would be sore for weeks! She had to be extremely careful with everything she did because her body broke down, wouldn't repair itself, or repaired very slowly. Hers was a rare and interesting case, because it wasn't like she was living in Africa—she lived in the United States and ate what appeared to be a good diet.

I also see many patients who have been diagnosed with multiple chemical sensitivities. These people are super sensitive to smells, perfumes, or any odor. Many can't have anything even touch their skin except for organic cotton or silk—synthetic fabrics make them break out in rashes, and they are hypersensitive to mold or pollens. It's a miserable existence. All of these patients are protein malnourished.

I also see many patients with fibromyalgia and chronic fatigue syndrome. All of them are protein malnourished.

All depressed people and people with anxiety are protein malnourished.

All osteoporotic patients are protein malnourished.

All patients with cancer are protein malnourished.

All patients with autoimmune diseases like Lupus and Rheumatoid Arthritis are protein malnourished.

All patients with sleep disorders are protein malnourished.

All Parkinson's patients are protein malnourished.

All Alzheimer's Dementia patients are protein malnourished.

Protein malnourishment is pervasive and is rarely looked for by medical doctors. It is treatable and can facilitate improvement in any of the above conditions. Keep in mind that essential amino acids are not the only nutrients the body needs; vitamins, minerals and essential fats at optimum levels are also necessary. When we treat a patient, we look for *all* deficiencies and work to replenish them. This is the first step of the secret to helping the chronically ill recover. The second step is dependent on the first; we must fix the deficiencies before we can get the accumulated toxins out of the body and complete the recovery process.

AMINO-FOCUSED NUTRITION

To give an example that contrasts from the ones above, but to further make the point, another patient of mine was one of the medical personnel for all of Lance Armstrong's pro cycling teams, during his now-tainted run of Tour de France victories. The team budgets were large enough to provide riders with everything they needed, including a traveling chef who made high-energy meals for them throughout the three-week race. The chef, along with the team doctors, did everything they could to improve the riders' nutrition-related performance and bring home a win.

As you can imagine, by the end of the Tour, the riders are broken down, tired, and in pain. After all, they fought through twenty-one intense, four or five hour rides on bikes at high altitudes. During one race season, the top-tier riders took Perfect Amino in large doses in addition to their regular diet. At the end of the Tour, their physician told me those riders weren't beaten down; they actually left the race in better shape than when they started. Their extraordinary daily recovery and increased strength makes it evident that if you give the body what it needs, especially essential amino acids in the right quantities, it can efficiently heal from maximum-trauma events.

It's common for patients who compete in triathlons or marathons to come down with a cold within a week after a race, because the body has limited resources for repair. It has a choice to make following such trauma, and it will usually prioritize healing of the heart, muscles, tendons, and ligaments ahead of the immune system. When intense skeletal repair is required, the immune system is depleted of its resources and will become weak. This leads to the onset of an upper respiratory infection or sometimes worse. However, if athletes load up on Perfect Amino a couple of days before and after an event, they usually won't come down with a cold. This is because there are enough essential amino acids to suffice for skeletal recovery and immune protection. I have validated this many times in my training and racing and with many other athletes that I work or train with.

The recovery needs of an athlete also apply to someone who has heart bypass surgery, or gets hit by a car: there is a high level of trauma and the body needs optimal protein nutrition to heal. If you provide the right kinds of amino acids, repair and healing will happen much faster.

My personal recovery time during training is greatly influenced by an adequate, amino acid-based diet. I have a very full schedule with training and my professional life, and many people ask how I'm able to do it—I get up at 5:20 a.m. and go to bed at 11:30 p.m. The answer is simple: I know how the body works and how to provide the nutrition it needs to perform and respond at the level of a thirty-year-old.

COMBATTING CHEMICAL TRAUMA

In addition to physical wear and tear, we live in environments where chemical trauma is a reality—we're constantly exposed to radiation, Wi-Fi, pesticides, chemicals, heavy metals, and drugs. All of these are toxic in that they produce free radicals that cause injury to structures of the body. This requires the body to continually repair the inner-lining cells of the blood vessels, neurons, and all exposed tissues with specialized protein enzymes needed for the job. This is a twenty-four-hour-a-day process. Our bodies weren't designed to handle this type of stress, and when they can't recover from this trauma, we develop chemical imbalances, and depression and brain fog can occur as a result. In fact, those imbalances are the main cause of aging.

If you've ever set foot into a sporting goods or home goods store, you may have experienced a sore throat or general feeling of being "out of it," from high levels of rubber and plastic chemical residues that off-gas from the products and fill the air. With adequate nutrition from organic Paleo type food and supplements of essential amino acids, your ability to deal with this exposure is much higher, no matter the environment.

CELLS IN REPAIR

Our bodies are structured to limit cell exposure to toxins via the intestines. They work to prevent those toxins from entering the bloodstream or penetrating the blood barrier around the brain. The intricate membranes surrounding our brains are designed to keep toxins out and protect internal cells, because if your brain goes bad, your body is in trouble.

In a normally functioning intestine, the mucosal inner cell lining will turn over every three or four days. In a protein-deficient person, however, turnover may take up to ten days and culminate in what is called a *leaky gut*: a malfunctioning gut membrane that "leaks" in what it shouldn't and won't absorb what it should. To better illustrate this, think of a fresh cut on your finger. It might close in three or four days, but for some other people, it might never fully heal. This could be due to poor circulation, and healing nutrients are unable to reach the finger. Similarly, you might eat healthy food on a regular basis, but if your gut isn't absorbing the nutrients, it's all for naught. Likewise, our pulmonary and intestinal membrane barriers are there to prevent the entry of noxious, foreign particles into the body—they work to keep your inner environment safe. They all have a high turnover rate, so fresh, healthy cells should be there to act as a barrier. In a protein malnourished person, the cellular integrity breaks down and one is susceptible to leaky membranes of the gut, lungs, and blood-brain barrier.

PROTEIN METABOLISM 101

Protein foods include meat, fish, eggs, beans, dairy products and amino acid mixtures from plants—so-called "plant proteins." The first thing that happens through chewing is that the proteins get broken down into smaller sizes where they enter the stomach, where Phase One of protein digestion begins.

The anatomy of a protein consists of a long string of linked amino acids, which are molecules made of carbon, hydrogen, oxygen, and nitrogen. There are twenty-two different ways that amino acids are configured for use in our body. If you imagine twenty-two different colored and shaped beads, each one unique, and all put together in a very exact order, that is what a protein looks like. When this chain hits the stomach, the acid level secreted by the stomach cells produces a chemical reaction that uncoils the protein. Then, an enzyme called *pepsin* starts breaking the bonds between the amino acids, and the chains split apart.

The following graphic is the basic template for an amino acid. The amino is the "N" (the nitrogen portion on the left side), and the acid portion is the COOH on the right side. The "R" may contain other molecules that make the twenty-two amino acids different in structure.

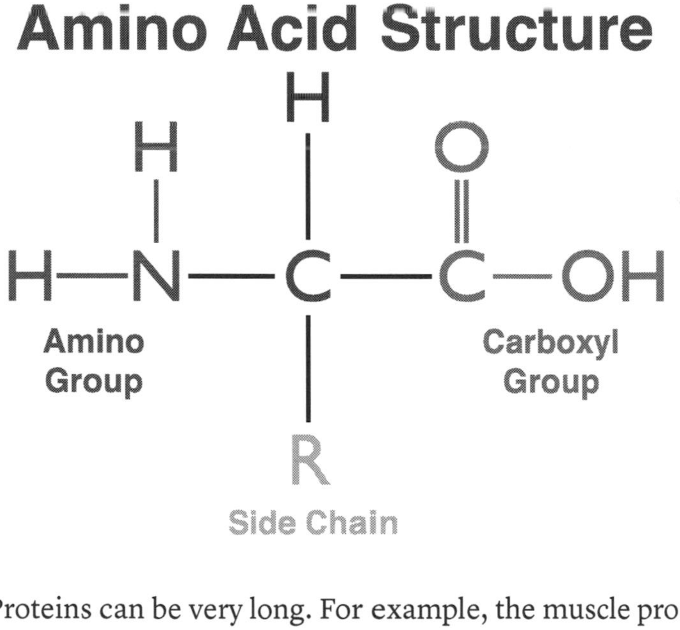

Amino Acid Structure

$$H-N-C-C-OH$$

Amino Group

Carboxyl Group

Side Chain

Proteins can be very long. For example, the muscle protein, actin, has six-thousand one hundred amino acids per chain. Here are some other proteins and the number of amino acids that make them.

Proteins and Functions

Protein	Function	Number of amino acids
Insulin	enzyme for sugar metabolism	51
Cytochrome c	enzyme for cell respiration	104
Growth Hormone	used in anti-aging treatment	191
Hemoglobin	oxygen transport to blood	574
Hexokinase	enzyme for glycolysis	730
Gamma Globulin	part of immune system in blood	1320
Actin	muscle action	6100

Modified from: Seager & Slabaugh, *Organic and Biochemistry for Today,* 4th ed, Brooks/Cole (2000)

Here is an example of what one of the proteins, insulin, looks like in three dimensions:

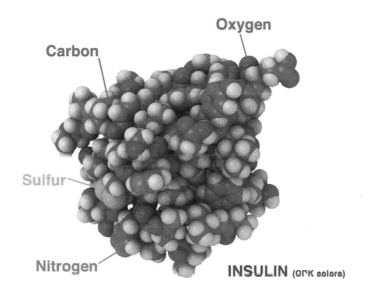

Carbon · Oxygen · Sulfur · Nitrogen · INSULIN (CPK colors)

There is a lot of breaking apart required in the process of digestion—it's the splitting of longer complex molecules into simpler ones by chemical means. After the partially digested proteins leave the stomach, they enter the small intestine where enzymes from the pancreas break the chains down further into individual amino acids.

When this long chain of amino acids is broken down into single amino acids, protein digestion is complete, and Phase Two can begin: they can then be absorbed by the intestinal cells and enter the bloodstream. Those individual amino acids are carried to our cells—they are actively brought into the cell where the process of protein synthesis can begin. For a muscle cell, it must put the amino acids back together one-by-one into a human muscle fiber called *myosin*, with six-thousand one hundred amino acids per single fiber, and three hundred seventy-four amino acids in the other portion of the muscle cell, *actin*. What a job!

Here is what the structure of every muscle fiber looks like. The following graphic shows the components of actin and myosin and how they come together from a relaxed to contracted state.

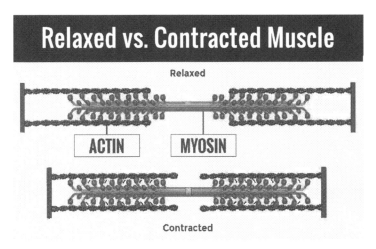

To give another example, let's look at the proteins that are part of every cell membrane in the body. If these proteins can't be manufactured due to amino acid deficiency, they will not function properly. They include transport proteins that move molecules in and out of the cell, docking proteins where outside molecules attach to give information to the cell, adhesion proteins where molecules can stick to the surface of the cell to cause change, etc.

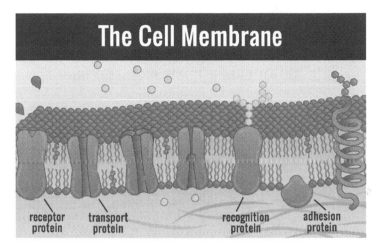

The Cell Membrane

receptor protein transport protein recognition protein adhesion protein

As you can see this process is unbelievably complicated. The miracle of life is incomprehensible. This process occurs in *every cell, every minute of the day* in the 100 trillion cells of the body, for the fifty-thousand different proteins that *make up* the body. However, the process can stall at any point. If someone lacks quality protein in their diet with too few, or an imbalance of essential amino acids, or has no stomach acid due to taking a drug to block it, they will have poor protein digestion. Pepsin only works when the acidity of the stomach is very low, with a pH of 1 to 2.

If there are not enough enzymes in the stomach or pancreas, or, a weak intestinal membrane from protein deficiency, then absorption will not occur—there is a catch-22 built into every cycle. Take the example of a gluten-sensitive person: a gluten sensitive person eats gluten, which causes degeneration in the intestinal membrane. The membrane then can't absorb nutrients efficiently, meaning it can't heal. And if you can't heal, you can't absorb. It's like the old rhyme, "for lack a nail the shoe was lost, for lack of shoe the soldier was lost, for lack of a soldier the battle was lost, for lack of battle the war was lost—all because a nail was lost."

	HEALTHY	DAMAGED
Duodenum		
Ileum		

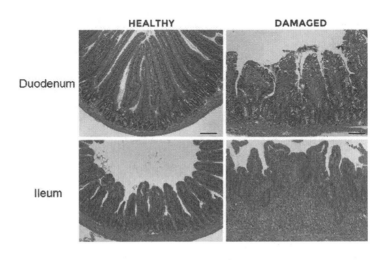

In the production of a protein made up of hundreds of amino acids, if any of the essential amino acid levels are low, the protein production will be stopped. It can't skip amino acid and go on to the next. That protein is just not produced, and the protein synthesis stops right there. If nutrition is not adequate, it could take days for that muscle fiber to be repaired or made—giving you a sore back for an entire week after chopping wood, for example. Or, if you are lacking the essential amino acid tryptophan and not making enough of the neurotransmitter serotonin, it can make depression linger on and on.

What Can Occur with Insufficient Protein

- Decreased body protein turnover
- Immune impairment
- Decreased organ mass
- Muscle wasting
- Connective tissue loss
- Bone loss
- Lower neurotransmitters
- Delayed healing
- Loss of training effect in athletes/ injury
- Lowered Hormones
- Lower enzyme levels with reduced liver detoxification, reduced ATP production, etc.

WHAT IS AN ESSENTIAL AMINO ACID?

At this point I want to clarify the term *Essential Amino Acid*.

Of the twenty-two amino acids that the body uses to make proteins, eight of them are classified as *essential*. This means that we must get these from food or supplements, because the body is unable to make them. If the body has the eight essential amino acids in the proper quantities and in the right proportion, then it can make the remaining fourteen non-essential acids. This is important because more than 50 percent of most proteins are made of these essential ones.

Essential Amino Acids

Methionine   Leucine   Isoleucine   Phenylalanine

Lysine   Valine   Threonine   Tryptophan

When the pancreatic cells get enough of the eight essential amino acids, they can make the protein insulin, which consists of two chains: thirty-one amino acids in one, and twenty in the other. All of the critical enzymes needed for energy, repair, detoxification, and growth are proteins made of amino acids. This allows the thyroid to make thyroid hormone, the pituitary to make growth hormone, etc.

Some textbooks will state that there are not just eight essential amino acids, but nine or ten, to include histidine and arginine. The argument is that young, growing children or the elderly require these additional two. Experiments have proven that when the eight essential amino acids are given in the right balance and quantity, the blood levels of the additional amino acids, histidine and arginine, will rise within a short time, proving that the body can make them, and they are not needed from an outside source.

AMINO ACID PATHWAYS

Within the cell, there are two pathways for amino acids. The first is called the *anabolic pathway*. Anabolic means "building up." It's the growth and creation of something big from something small—it is the building of proteins from amino acids. In the anabolic pathway, the amino acids that are eaten, digested, absorbed, and reached the cell are then made into a protein. That could be a hormone, an enzyme, a neurotransmitter, or a piece of hair. This pathway takes the raw materials (amino acids) and makes them into proteins.

The other pathway is called the *catabolic pathway*. Catabolic means "breaking down" or "breaking apart." It takes the complex and makes it simpler. When the amino acid gets to the cell and it is not needed for protein synthesis, the cell will break it down into molecules of carbon, hydrogen, and oxygen—these are carbohydrates and can be used as fuel. The other molecule that results from the breakdown of an amino acid is nitrogen. This is toxic waste and must be processed by the body into *urea*, a protein waste product that is excreted mostly in the urine. The *blood urea nitrogen* test (BUN) is a measure of the amount of nitrogen that is processed down the catabolic pathway.

You've probably heard that protein is equivalent to four calories per gram. This is only true if the amino acid goes down the catabolic pathway and results in a carbohydrate, which can be burned as fuel or stored as glycogen (for later use as a fuel), and the leftover nitrogen gets dumped. If the amino acid goes down the anabolic pathway and it becomes a structural or another type of protein, it is *not* burned and is not worth any calories.

Another very interesting piece of information can be understood from this and is a discovery of considerable magnitude. When predicting protein nutritional value, it's only *the amount of essential amino acids (EAA)* and their relative values that determine whether the protein will be "processed" down the anabolic or catabolic pathway. (About 50 percent or more of most body proteins are made of EAA, the major exception to this being collagen because it has no tryptophan and is mostly composed of four nonessential amino acids.)

FOR GEEKS ONLY

If we did a balance study and measured how many grams of nitrogen a person was fed (remember that carbs and fats have no nitrogen) and we collected urine to see how many grams of nitrogen came out (catabolized amino acids yielding free nitrogen), we could calculate a new value known as AMINO ACID UTILIZATION (AAU). The formula is **grams of nitrogen out divided by grams of nitrogen in** to yield a percentage of AAU. For the calculation, most proteins are about 16 percent nitrogen by weight, so we use **.16** to determine the grams of nitrogen taken in.

For example, if you ate sixty grams of steak protein, and that was your only protein for the day, the formula would be 60 X .16 = 9.6. This is the number of grams of nitrogen that you took in. Then, if we collected all of your urine from that day, we could use it to calculate the percentage of nitrogen that was retained from that protein, giving us the AAU. That formula is grams of nitrogen out/grams of nitrogen in = AAU.

High-quality proteins have a high AAU and low-quality ones have a lower one. AAU gives us a way to measure which dietary proteins our bodies can best utilize to make and repair our body proteins.

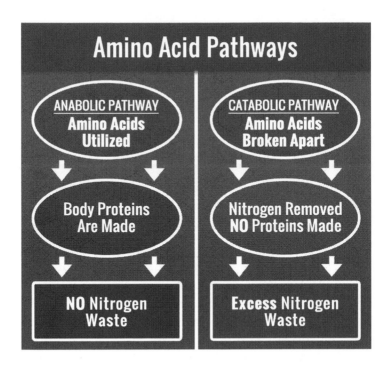

Once the amino acids reach the cell they are either taken down an anabolic (building) pathway and formed into body proteins, such as enzymes, collagen, hemoglobin, neurotransmitters, or the catabolic (breaking down) pathway where they result in a carbon-hydrogen-oxygen chain plus nitrogen waste. There are no storage pools for nitrogen, so it goes to the liver where it is turned into urea and is then excreted mainly through the urine.

THE DYSFUNCTIONAL CAR FACTORY

The following is an analogy of how nitrogen waste is processed:

Let's say you work in a car factory, and the minimum parts required to complete a fully functioning car are:

1. a chassis
2. four wheels
3. a motor
4. a steering wheel

There is a mix up in the ordering of these materials, and one hundred chassis, one hundred motors, one hundred wheels, and one steering wheel arrive at the factory. At that point, how many cars can you make at the factory? Only one. In addition, the factory has no storage space for the extra parts and you must get rid of them.

This is similar to what happens in the human body with the consumption of proteins. Each protein, whether it be from a vegetable or animal source is made up of from tens to thousands of amino acids. Many of them are not the ones that are needed by the cell at the moment they arrive. The cell has no storage depot for amino acids, and the unnecessary ones are quickly shunted down the catabolic pathway.

Since the most valuable amino acids are the essential ones, the body will take them and turn them into proteins *if* there are adequate amounts to make the given protein that the cell is working on. In very technical experiments, it was found that there is an ideal ratio of the essential amino acids, such that all of the amino acids can be utilized for protein synthesis. This means that almost no nitrogen waste is produced, less than one percent becomes calories, and nearly all of the aminos become protein. This gives us an amino acid utilization of 99 percent, which is the Perfect Amino formula. There are only four calories in ten grams of Perfect Amino and virtually no free-nitrogen waste.

AMINO ACID UTILIZATION OF VARIOUS PROTEINS

If we compare other proteins and their amino acid utilization we find the following:

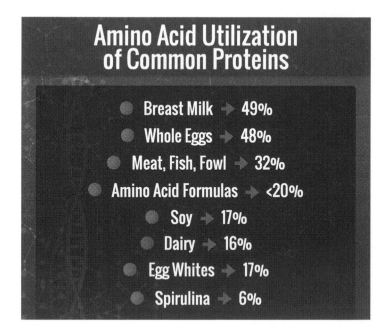

Amino Acid Utilization of Common Proteins

- Breast Milk → 49%
- Whole Eggs → 48%
- Meat, Fish, Fowl → 32%
- Amino Acid Formulas → <20%
- Soy → 17%
- Dairy → 16%
- Egg Whites → 17%
- Spirulina → 6%

If we consider whey protein, only 16 percent of the amino acids are used for protein synthesis. That means 84 percent becomes calories that are turned into sugar. Whey protein is known to be insulinogenic—it's like taking a hit of sugar for your body. Despite its positive commercial presence as a protein, whey is more utilized as a carb, meaning it can cause weight gain, or cause fat to remain in a static state instead of being burned.

The beauty of Perfect Amino is that it's a mixture of the eight essential amino acids with an ideal ratio of one to another. Since this ideal balance is being met, less than 1 percent of it is turned into nitrogen waste. Nearly all of it is used to make protein—and that's what our cells want!

THE IMPORTANCE OF BASIC PROTEIN KNOWLEDGE

As stated earlier, the structure of our bodies and its enzyme systems are made of protein. Bones by weight are about 40 percent collagen, which is a protein. Organs, connective tissue, digestion, and enzymes for energy production are also protein-based, along with neurotransmitters and many hormones. Armed with that knowledge alone, we know that inadequate amounts of essential amino acids drastically affect the structure of the body and its overall function.

As an example, we find many patients with low *chymotrypsin* (CHYMO). This is the major pancreatic enzyme responsible for protein digestion and can be measured through a stool sample. A patient with low CHYMO can't digest protein very well, which leaves them undigested, and thus unavailable to the cells to make new proteins or repair damaged ones. We've seen CHYMO levels in patients rise after taking Perfect Amino, which then allows more complete protein digestion and more amino acids for the cells. This leads to faster-healing wounds, improved moods, sleep patterns, and higher energy.

To give another example, patients with low levels of thyroid hormone often have low levels of *tyrosine*, the amino acid that is made into thyroid hormone. To make thyroid hormone the body adds three or four iodine molecules to it. This requires specialized enzymes (proteins) to do this. The process also requires the presence of enough iodine, selenium, zinc, vitamin C, and magnesium. The body makes tyrosine from an essential amino acid called *phenylalanine*. When there are adequate amounts of this essential amino acid, the levels of tyrosine will also be adequate. Replenishing amino acids (and the other factors mentioned above) can improve thyroid function, and eventually, patients may be able to stop taking thyroid hormone altogether because the body now has the raw materials to synthesize it.

Now you understand how human physiology works in the process of digestion and what is needed to maintain good health. Since protein nutrition is the key to these processes, you need to know what's true and what's false about protein. I'll reveal the truth behind some common myths in the next chapter, so you can make informed decisions about your protein intake.

CHAPTER TWO

PROTEIN MYTHS

Several common myths surround protein and its importance in our lives. This chapter offers insight into the problems created by these myths and how to approach solving them.

PROTEIN MYTH ONE: ALL PROTEINS ARE THE SAME.

You may think there's nothing wrong with this statement, but one look at this amino acid utilization chart shows us that they are most definitely *not* the same. The chart shows the substances and foods people consider to be sources of protein and their utilization rates based on amino acid profiles.

Nutritional Value: Dietary Protein

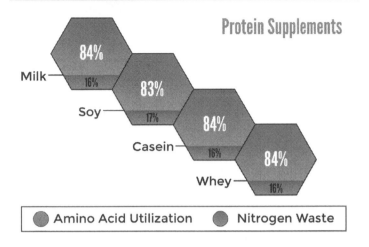

Protein Supplements

Milk — 84% / 16%
Soy — 83% / 17%
Casein — 84% / 16%
Whey — 84% / 16%

● Amino Acid Utilization   ● Nitrogen Waste

Let's consider algae for a moment. Many health food stores are big on selling spirulina, a popular and nutritious algae. A common sales line touts it as one of Earth's primary foods, which is true, as spirulina is packed with minerals, phytonutrients, and essential fatty acids. People who sell algae say this wonder food is great for building bodies because it can build and sustain the life of a whale.

But don't rush to your local health food store's algae aisle just yet. The balance of the eight essential amino acids in a food must be exact—if even one of the essential amino acids is low, it throws the entire nutritional profile off balance. Spirulina is deficient in the essential amino acids lysine and methionine to the point that the utilization is calculated at 6 percent or less in some twenty-four examined species. It's definitely a good source of green food, but it's not a valuable source of protein.

The next time you look at the side of a yogurt carton and it says 14 grams of protein, be aware that only 16 percent is usable. A Balance Bar has 14 grams of dairy and soy protein, but only 16 percent is usable. And a can of tuna fish has 16 grams of protein, of which 33 percent is usable. Please refer to the chart for more information.

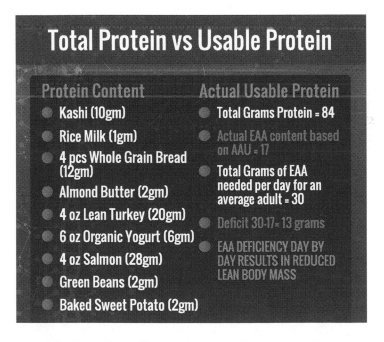

Total Protein vs Usable Protein

Protein Content	Actual Usable Protein
Kashi (10gm)	Total Grams Protein = 84
Rice Milk (1gm)	Actual EAA content based on AAU = 17
4 pcs Whole Grain Bread (12gm)	Total Grams of EAA needed per day for an average adult = 30
Almond Butter (2gm)	
4 oz Lean Turkey (20gm)	
6 oz Organic Yogurt (6gm)	Deficit 30-17= 13 grams
4 oz Salmon (28gm)	EAA DEFICIENCY DAY BY DAY RESULTS IN REDUCED LEAN BODY MASS
Green Beans (2gm)	
Baked Sweet Potato (2gm)	

Don't believe that all proteins are all the same, because they aren't! This leads us to the next myth that permeates the dietary industry, with dieticians included.

PROTEIN MYTH TWO: PEOPLE ARE GETTING ENOUGH PROTEIN IN THEIR DAILY LIVES.

Through my years of testing and reviewing essential amino acid levels of patients, I can tell you that countless people aren't getting enough protein. This issue is not made apparent by physical appearance; at first glance of these three images, most people assume the obese man certainly isn't protein malnourished. However, the fact is, *all three probably are*. Many obese and starving people are protein malnourished, but so are people with "normal" diets—it all comes down to essential amino acid levels in the blood.

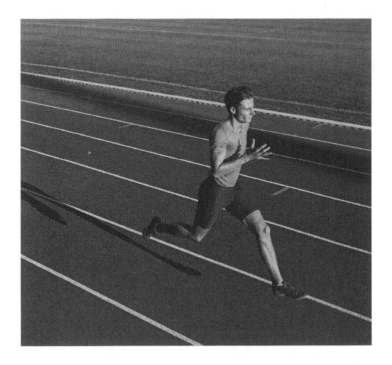

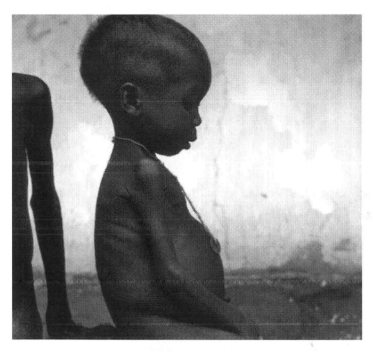

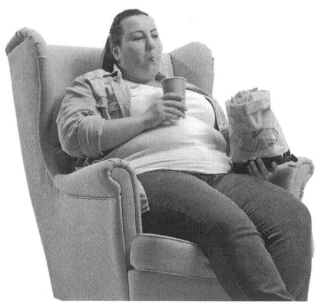

Dieticians offer the blanket belief that daily intake of one gram of protein per body weight is adequate nourishment—this generalization assumes that *all* proteins are the same. This concept is flawed and contributes to the widespread belief of this myth. Athletes, pregnant women, and those recovering from injury or surgery need more protein than the average person. These people need to consume more than the recommended amount of protein to provide their bodies with what they need. This belief also assumes that they chew their food adequately; have enough stomach acid and pepsin in their stomachs; have sufficient pancreatic enzymes; the lining cells of their intestine can absorb the digested food; the lining cells have not been compromised due to glyphosate damaging their membrane; their membranes are also intact after eating foods they are allergic to (like gluten); and they have no parasites, yeasts, or bad bacteria that are living there and causing damage to the membrane. These assumptions are made but *never* looked into by the vast majority of medical doctors, nutritionists or dieticians.

Everyone needs clean protein sources in adequate amounts, and more importantly, we must be able to digest and absorb it. Digestion can be a challenge for many people, and supplements are required in those cases. I'm definitely not suggesting that people *only* take essential amino acid tablets or drink a special elixir for their protein source, but high-quality protein with the addition of supplements can greatly improve a person's health.

PROTEIN MYTH THREE: SOY IS A GOOD SOURCE OF PROTEIN.

Earlier, we discussed popular misconceptions about whey and spirulina. Both are viewed in a favorable light and soy is, too. However, soy rides the popularity roller coaster just like every other food in the area of diet science—and right now, it's very much out of favor. It's known as a source of protein in terms of its amino acid content and utilization, but the truth is that soy is very similar to whey.

PROTEIN MYTH FOUR: COLLAGEN IS A GOOD SOURCE OF PROTEIN.

Collagen is the most prevalent protein in the human body, making up about 30 percent of all body proteins. There has been a big rise in the popularity of promoting collagen as an ideal protein supplement, and it's now available in powder form for protein shakes and soup mixes, in nutritional bars, and even face creams. With all of these products on the market, one might think that eating collagen is a great source of this protein. However, we need to look more closely at this logic and ask if their claims are true.

When we look at the amino acid profile of collagen, over

50 percent comes from four *nonessential* amino acids: proline, glycine, hydroxyproline and arginine. Collagen is missing the essential amino acid tryptophan and is deficient in three other essential amino acids: isoleucine, threonine, and methionine[3].

It has been proven that if a dietary protein is missing any of the essential amino acids, the body is unable to utilize it as a precursor for protein synthesis. If we did an analysis for amino acid utilization (AAU), then collagen would be at zero percent because essential amino acids are missing. Compare that to 99 percent AAU for Perfect Amino.

The body can absorb the amino acids from collagen if it is eaten along with other foods that can make up for lack of tryptophan and low amounts of isoleucine, threonine, and methionine—however, the AAU will still be very low. This means that most of the collagen you eat will end up as sugar or carbs, and to boot, there will be a heavy burden of nitrogen to detox. This is disappointing in light of the marketing surrounding collagen products, but it's the truth—you'll have a much better AAU if you eat steak, chicken, fish or eggs.

---

3   Scott, Trudy, "Collagen and gelatin lower serotonin: does this increase your anxiety and depression," Every woman over 29 blog, September 29, 2017, https://www.everywomanover29. com/blog/collagen-gelatin-lower-serotonin-increase-anxiety-depression/

Also, you'll want to be cautious if you purchase and use collagen products. They contain collagen from animal tissues—joints, bones, skin, hair, feathers, hooves from cows and pigs, or fish. These animals may or may not have been grass fed, free of antibiotics or hormones, or free of GMO feed unless stated by the manufacturer. Recent testing reveals that popular collagen and bone broth products contain a number of potentially hazardous contaminants, including antibiotics, prescription drug metabolites, parabens, steroids, and insecticides.[4][5]

PROTEIN MYTH FIVE: BRANCHED CHAIN AMINO ACIDS ARE GOOD FOR MUSCLE RECOVERY.

Branched chain amino acids (BCAAs) are heavily promoted for athletic recovery and building muscle protein. BCAAs include leucine, isoleucine, and valine. These are three of the eight essential amino acids, but since five essentials are missing, they also have an AAU value of zero percent. You can't make any proteins with just three amino acids—all eight are required at the same time, in the right proportions for maximum AAU.

---

4   Marshall, Lisa, "Collagen: 'Fountain of Youth' or Edible Hoax?" webmd.com, March 8, 2018, https://www.webmd.com/skin-problems-and-treatments/news/20180308/collagen-supplements-what-the-research-shows

5   mercola.com, "Buyer Beware: Most Collagen Supplements Sourced from CAFOs, October 23, 2017, https://articles.mercola.com/sites/articles/archive/2017/10/23/nonorganic-collagen-products.aspx

Even though their AAU is zero percent, BCAAs are not useless. There is evidence that if your body is short of carbs and starts to break down muscle for calories, it will use the BCAAs for fuel instead of pirating its own proteins. So, it does have a muscle sparing effect, but you could also eat a banana and get the same result.

PROTEIN MYTH SIX: EGG WHITES ARE A GOOD SOURCE OF PROTEIN.

As I mentioned earlier, whole eggs—the white plus the yolk—are the best source of dietary protein, with the exception of breast milk. And since breast milk is not readily available, we look to eggs for protein. Eggs have an AAU of 48 percent and are a cut above meats, fish or any dairy proteins.

Some people are convinced that they should not eat egg yolks due to concerns about cholesterol. This is a totally incorrect assumption, as it has never been proven that eating eggs contributes to plaque buildup in the arteries.

However, many cardiologists have been brainwashed with this theory, and they dutifully pass it on—their patients think they should avoid egg yolks, or only eat two eggs a week, or some such propaganda. So, they resort to eating egg whites.

The truth is, without the yolk, eggs are no longer the best source of dietary protein—they become more like dairy or soybeans and have a low AAU of 16 percent. Egg yolks contain the essential amino acid methionine, and you should not deprive yourself of it. So, eat your eggs as nature intended: with the yolks. And enjoy them without limit!

THE WHOLE TRUTH

The amount of misinformation that exists around nutrition and nutritional "science" is truly amazing. The bottom line is that if you look at profiles of serum blood amino acid levels, you will come to the conclusion that our bodies don't get, digest, or absorb enough protein. Even when we think we eat enough protein throughout the day, the utilization rate is low, and I'm revealing the truth behind these myths to explain that most people are protein malnourished. Simply put, we need access to adequate amounts of clean protein, and we need to properly digest and absorb it. We'll talk more about how the body digests protein in the chapters to come.

CHAPTER THREE

ARE WE PROTEIN MALNOURISHED?

Between 2.5 million and ten thousand years ago, Paleolithic Era man obtained much of their protein from game, fish, and eggs. At that time, animals roamed free and pollution wasn't a concern, so the overall nutritional health of humans was at a high level. If we still ate food like our hunter-gatherer ancestors did, there would be no need for protein or vitamin or mineral supplementation.

Things changed about ten thousand years ago at the dawn of the Neolithic Era, when humans settled into communities, began farming, and domesticated animals. In our modern-day era, they are fed GMO corn and soybeans that are laced with toxic herbicides like Roundup. These modern methods have caused plants, animals, and much of the soil to become highly polluted over time and ultimately created the problem we face today: a lack of clean protein sources.

The steak we eat most likely comes from cows that ate genetically-modified organisms (GMOs) and glyphosate-saturated corn. High-end steakhouses often tout "corn-fed beef" as a delicacy, as if corn is the cow's natural food! Not only that, but they were probably given artificial hormones to fatten them up before slaughter and antibiotics throughout their entire lives. The meat is then processed, placed on Styrofoam pads, and wrapped in cellophane. These packaging practices significantly increase the levels of toxic chemicals (like phthalates) contained in the food. It's a formidable challenge today to obtain clean, healthy food, but it's equally as challenging to find food that isn't packaged in toxic materials.

TO CHARBROIL OR NOT TO CHARBROIL?

We don't just need to be cautious about how our food is packaged—we also need to take into consideration how our food is prepared. Personally, I like the taste of charbroiled meat, but the burning produces carcinogens. A million years ago, people cooked over fires and burned their meat all the time, but they also weren't exposed to other chemicals. In today's world with its plethora of harmful substances, gobbling a hunk of charred meat carves another notch on the poor nutrition wall—and there are only so many notches until the body breaks down.

THE SCOURGE OF POLLUTED PROTEIN

It's nearly impossible to go to most grocery stores today and find non-polluted protein sources. The "mass manufacturing" of chicken, fish, milk, eggs, and other foods focuses on quick, convenient, low-cost production.

When left to their own devices, chickens wander freely and eat grubs and worms, but modern-day poultry breeders raise them in a controlled environment. Nearly every modern commercial egg farm keeps chickens in small cages. Lights stay on for long hours so the birds believe it's daytime, encouraging them to produce the maximum amount of eggs possible; farmers feed them grain meal, and they never roam free or see the outside world.

Some companies claim to sell pastured eggs, but they stretch that term to its limits. They keep the chickens in a barn with a small door—the birds don't go outside because they can't find the door or get through it, but the eggs are still labeled as "pastured." Now, there are companies that adhere to sound production processes and make genuinely healthy products, but the sad fact is that a high percentage of the food packaged in modern countries is polluted.

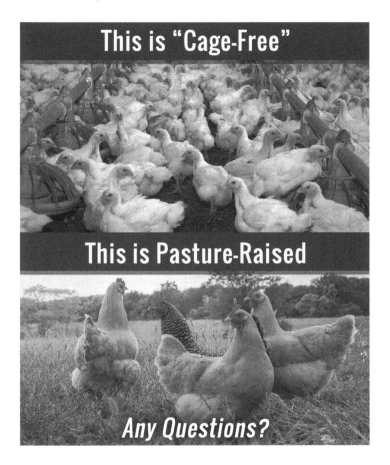
This is "Cage-Free"

This is Pasture-Raised

Any Questions?

IS THERE HOPE FOR CHANGE?

There is good news in the midst of this problem: change is coming. However, there is also some bad news: the change is very slow and faces powerful foes. The American population is becoming more informed regarding food production practices, and they're beginning to use their dollars to vote for cleaner food. Some people choose to be vegan or vegetarian and avoid meat altogether, but that does nothing to solve the external problem.

Big Agriculture and Big Pharma have an enormous influence on the government. The current head of the U.S. Department of Agriculture is a former Monsanto executive. (If you're familiar with the name, you know it's one of the most powerful chemical companies in the world.) I find it interesting that while former President Barack Obama spoke openly about healthy food and a healthy lifestyle, he appointed a chemical executive to lead our country's agricultural efforts.

If you watch a grocery check-out line for an hour and see what people are buying, it's no wonder we're sick. Soda, chemicalized and glyphosate-laden cereals, fast food, frozen meals, contaminated meats, and everything in plastic is producing a race of suboptimal people.

Nabisco		
Ritz Crackers		Glyphosate - 270.24 ppb
Triscuit Crackers		Glyphosate - 89.68 ppb
Oreo Original		Glyphosate - 289.47* ppb
Oreo Double Stuf Chocolate Sandwich Cookies		Glyphosate - 140.90* ppb
Oreo Double Stuf Golden Sandwich Cookies		Glyphosate - 215.40* ppb
PepsiCo		
Stacy's Simply Naked Pita Chips (Frito-Lay)		Glyphosate - 812.53 ppb
Lay's Kettle Cooked Original		Glyphosate - 452.71* ppb
Doritos Cool Ranch		Glyphosate - 481.27* ppb
Fritos Original (100% Whole Grain)		Glyphosate - 174.71* ppb
Campbell Soup Company		
Goldfish Crackers Original (Pepperidge Farm)		Glyphosate - 18.40 ppb
Goldfish Crackers Colors		Glyphosate - 8.02 ppb
Goldfish Crackers (Whole Grain)		Glyphosate - 24.58 ppb
Little Debbie		
Oatmeal Creme Pies		Glyphosate - 264.28* ppb
Lucy's		
Oatmeal Cookies (Gluten-Free)		Glyphosate - 452.44* ppb
Whole Foods		
365 Organic Golden Round Crackers**		Glyphosate - 119.12* ppb
Back to Nature		
Crispy Cheddar Crackers		Glyphosate - 327.22* ppb

Limit of Quantitation: 5 ppb

* Theses examples exhibit very low/and or response. The amounts listed above are rough estimates at best, and may not be a fully accurate representation of the sample.

* Widespread contamination in food supply - even organic crops have been found to be contaminated.

The above graphic was inspired by graphic variations published in multiple articles by: www.foodbabe.com, www.raisevegan.com, and www.mamavation.com. Information regarding the levels of glyphosate in popular food brands can be found on the Environmental Working Group website at: https://www.ewg.org

The only way to put a wrench in the works is to simply stop buying polluted foods. I believe people can and will change if they care about their health and are determined enough to make a difference.

THE DISAPPEARANCE OF A HEALTHY PEOPLE

During my pediatric residency in 1978 at the University of California Hospital in San Diego, the renowned and respected department chairman, Dr. William Nyhan M.D., made rounds with us once a week. I remember we visited a little fifteen-month-old one day, and he said, "When we're done with rounds today, each of you should come back and examine this child. You'll probably never see another one like him in your career. He has autism."

According to him, the incidence of autism at the time was roughly one in 150,000—he told us that a busy pediatrician over a forty-year career would never see that many patients—indicating that the odds of encountering an autistic child were extremely rare.

Today, the autism rate is roughly one in every forty children.[6] Unfortunately, it's not genetic, it's not an accident, and it's not getting better—I believe this a real epidemic. If this trend continues, in twenty-five years millions of the population will be on disability, and many more children will have special needs due to the dire effect of our food and toxic environment. The main purpose of this book is to educate you about protein and discuss Perfect Amino, but its secondary purpose is to give you a wake-up call.

---

6   Nedleman, Michael, "Autism prevalence now 1 in 40 U.S. kids, study estimates," cnn.com, November 26, 2018, https://www.cnn.com/2018/11/26/health/autism-prevalence-study/index.html

You must be careful with your lifestyle, and make wise choices regarding what you eat, and what you allow yourself to be exposed to.

Our bodies don't know what to do with the combinations of chemicals and substances in the environment that have never before been seen in human history. Thirty years ago, 25 percent of our children didn't have asthma. Now, in the first year of a child's life, they are injected with twenty-six different vaccines, many of which are laced with formaldehyde, aluminum, mercury, and dead animal parts. The mercury level in some of these vaccines is fifty thousand times greater than what is legally acceptable in drinking water, and they are often given to babies on the day of their birth![7] [8]

7   Geier, David A., Kern, Janet K., Hooker, Brian S., King, Paul G., Sykes, Lisa K., Geier, Mark R., "Thimerosal-Containing Hepatitis B Vaccination and the Risk for Diagnosed Specific Delays in Development in the United States: A Case-Control Study in the Vaccine Safety Datalink," North American Journal of Medical Sciences, October 6, 2014, https://www.ncbi.nlm.nih.gov/pmc/articles/PMC4215490/

8   Kirby, David, "Help the Environment, Get a Flu Shot," huffingtonpost.com, December 18, 2006, https://www.huffingtonpost.com/david-kirby/help-the-environment-get-_b_36604.html

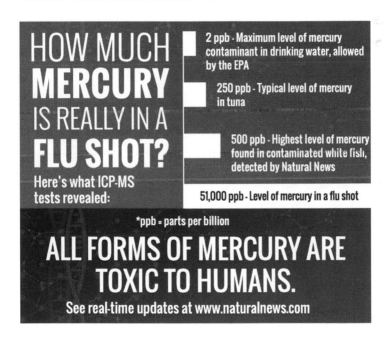

The health of our children is being devastated by cancer, ADD, autism, diabetes, and obesity. Pregnant mothers who haven't taken care of themselves are riddled with environmental poisons, and the fetus becomes a dumping ground for toxins—this results in many children coming into the world at a disadvantage.

THE CATASTROPHE OF GMO FOODS

We clearly see the impact of toxicity in modern-day schools, where food-allergic kids are segregated to peanut or dairy-free tables; we see it on flights that no longer serve peanuts because someone on board may be allergic. Tomatoes and other plants are genetically modified so they look pretty, last long, and are pesticide-tolerant, but the end result is food containing peanut genes or fish DNA—components that should never have been part of the food's makeup.

Genetically modifying foods also affects their taste. When you compare an organic, vine-ripened tomato to the "usual" one available in the grocery store, the organic one has a beautiful natural color and delicious flavor; whereas the modified one is faded red and tastes like sour cardboard!

THE SALVATION DIET CRAZE

There is a host of cure-all diets out there that are all the rage in fitness circles, dietician forums, and magazines. However, nearly every one of these diets lack adequate amounts of protein.

The Vegan Hallelujah diet, for example, consists entirely of vegetables, with very low amounts of protein; the same goes for the Gerson and China Study diets. Even the Standard American Diet (SAD) is often deficient in essential amino acids. These particular diets might be good for you in some respects since they're high in phytonutrients and fiber, but I've measured the blood amino acid levels in many patients who have been on those diets, and their levels are almost always lacking. They'll also feel tired and lose lean body mass due to lack of sufficient protein. Please refer to the charts for more information.

NUTRITION MADE SIMPLE

To make your nutritional life much less complicated, skip the fad diets and follow a Paleo-type food pattern that includes organic fruits and vegetables; grass-fed, hormone free, and antibiotic free meats; wild-caught fish; pastured, whole eggs, tree nuts, and seeds. And if you desire it, you can also eat organic butter and whole cream.

If weight loss is your goal, decreasing the amount of fruits and starchy vegetables is usually effective—this can help you achieve your ideal weight. Healthy oils like olive, avocado, coconut, butter, lard, or duck fat can be used liberally, but trans fats should be avoided. Most people can "cheat" on up to three meals per week, but we ask them to avoid gluten and processed foods as much as possible—if it comes in a box or a package and has unrecognizable ingredients, don't eat it. When people first start a nutritional program, I recommend that people don't consume any grains, legumes, nightshade vegetables, or alcohol for the first six weeks. After following this protocol, many report a decrease in bloating, heartburn and gas, and an improvement in energy, so they decide to continue eating this way, with the exception of special occasions.

Now that you understand the external factors that contribute to the protein problem—a lack of clean protein sources, toxins in our food, and misinformation surrounding popular diets—we'll move on to the internal factors that can inhibit protein digestion and absorption.

CHAPTER FOUR

BARRIERS TO PROTEIN DIGESTION AND ABSORPTION

As we've already discussed, access to clean protein sources is only one part of the problem; it must also be properly digested. This is a complicated process that requires a healthy gastrointestinal (GI) tract, which, unfortunately, many people lack.

You must absorb enough essential amino acids per pound or kilogram of body weight, because the protein we need is made from aminos. Like it or not, animal proteins are the best natural source of essential amino acids for our bodies to function optimally. Vegetable proteins, on the other hand, have mixes of essential amino acids, but they are lacking in one or two—they don't nourish as well as animal protein. In other words, the level of amino acid utilization is poor. The bottom line is that our body is an animal body, and it needs proteins from *animal foods* to maintain its lean body mass.

STOMACH ACID AT WORK

In Chapter One, we discussed how protein is digested by the body. Now, we'll take it a step further and talk about the role of stomach acid in this process. Ideally, protein digestion begins in the mouth—the process of chewing breaks the contents into a liquid so that stomach acids can chemically break down the fibers. (For the elderly, or for people who are missing teeth, this step is not completed and that can create a barrier to adequate protein digestion).

Once food reaches the stomach, the true digestion process commences. Stomach hydrochloric acid (HCl) is added to the liquid mixture of food, and the acids cause the protein's coiled structures to open up or uncoil. The HCl also activates the pepsinogen enzyme to its active form, which is called pepsin. Pepsin starts to separate the protein amino acid chains into smaller units. If a muscle fiber has 6100 amino acids per chain of myosin, then those chains are "chopped up" into much shorter ones.

For this process to occur, the acid levels in the stomach must be at the pH level of 1 to 2, which is very acidic.

We measure acidity and alkalinity by using the pH scale. The scale goes from 1 to 14. The lower the number the stronger the acid. In the middle is water which has a pH of about 7. This is considered neutral. Above 7 and up to 14 is alkaline. For the proteins to uncoil sufficiently and for the pepsinogen to be activated requires a pH of 1-2. Due to aging or nutritional deficiencies, most people over the age of forty have a stomach pH that is higher than the one-to-two range. Since digestion is compromised at higher pH levels, they won't digest protein as well as a twenty-year-old will.

For example, a strand of steak or halibut is a long muscle protein made up of thousands of amino acids per strand, and it must be broken down into smaller pieces until it hits the digestion endpoint in the small intestine, where all amino acids are either single, or in much shorter chains in order for them to be absorbed in the small intestine.

Stomach Acid
The Seven Major Functions

1) Sterilizes the food
2) Denatures or uncoils the protein

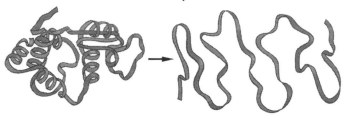

Active (functional) protein   Denatured protein

3) Pepsinogen activation to pepsin
4) Pepsin breaks down protein structure

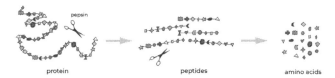

protein   peptides   amino acids

5) Activates intrinsic factor (so vitamin B12 can be absorbed)
6) Stimulates bile flow from liver and pancreatic enzymes to the small intestine
7) Closes the esophageal sphincter

Signs That You Have Low Stomach Acids

1) Gas and belching (from living bacteria ferments in the stomach)

2) GERD or acid reflux (due to open gastroesophageal junction)

3) Bloating and cramping (due to bacteria in stomach, small intestine carbohydrate ferments, and delayed opening of pyloric sphincter)

4) Nausea

5) Bad breath (due to fermentation in the stomach)

6) Undigested food present in stools

7) Dislike of animal proteins (due to inability to digest them properly)

8) Anemia (due to lack of protein digestion)

9) Weak fingernails and slow hair growth

10) Rosacea (red face, nose and cheek rash due to lack of stomach acid)

11) Fatigue (due to lack of HCl, causing poor mineral absorption)

12) Depression

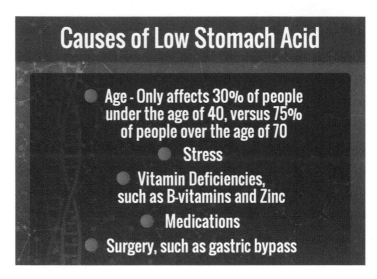

Causes of Low Stomach Acid

- Age - Only affects 30% of people under the age of 40, versus 75% of people over the age of 70
- Stress
- Vitamin Deficiencies, such as B-vitamins and Zinc
- Medications
- Surgery, such as gastric bypass

That said, there are roughly twenty-four million prescriptions written every month *in the United States,* with fifteen million for Nexium alone.[9] This number doesn't include all of the purchases of drugs that block stomach acid to relieve heartburn and acid reflux—billion-dollar brands like Zantac and Pepcid are available over-the-counter. These drugs poison the parietal cells in the stomach (the ones that make hydrochloric acid), so they will stop producing acid, which is detrimental to protein digestion among other things.

If the pH of the stomach reaches a level of seven, it fully compromises digestion and impairs mineral absorption—we often find that individuals with a high stomach pH

---

9   Science News, "Popular heartburn drugs linked to higher early death risk," Science Daily, July 5, 2017, https://www.sciencedaily.com/releases/2017/07/170705113546.htm

also have zinc, selenium, iron, iodine, and magnesium deficiencies. (Refer to the chart for more information).

Stomach pH also influences digestive system functionality. There is a valve between the esophagus and stomach called the *gastro esophageal sphincter* which is triggered to close when stomach acidity is high. If the pH is 1 or 2, the valve works as it should: it closes, and you won't get reflux. If you have a pH of 4 or 5, you're still acidic, but not enough to trigger the valve to close. This pH level causes acids to bubble up into your lower esophagus, which can cause burning in the throat, heartburn, and pain. (This is the typical mechanism of action in gastro esophageal reflux disease, or GERD).

If the cause of heartburn is lowered amounts of stomach acid, we give patients hydrochloric acid tablets to take with meals, which will lower the pH and close the valve— these tablets eliminate heartburn without the need for stomach acid-blocking drugs. If you suspect that you have this condition, you can work with your nutritional-oriented health care practitioner to monitor you for healing and the best results.

FOOD STERILITY AND US

The food we eat is not sterile, and we certainly don't make a habit of boiling everything before we eat it. We eat raw fruits and vegetables all the time, and some people even eat raw fish or meat! Our food is always contaminated with various bacteria, parasites, and sometimes fungi. Stomach acid is the body's main protection to stop those contaminants from reaching the small intestine—these foreign organisms are "boiled in acid" so to speak, so our body can defend against them.

When people take medications to deal with heartburn or GERD, this can put them at risk for bacteria, parasites and fungi. Without adequate stomach acid, these organisms can survive in the stomach and pass along to the small intestine where they can take up residence—this is known as *small intestinal bacterial overgrowth* or *SIBO*. Once they are there, they can cause inflammation of the small intestinal wall, which can compromise mineral and protein absorption. These foreign invaders can also ferment the food coming through the small and large intestines, which can lead to the production of methane and other gases, causing bloating and abdominal discomfort. In addition, these organisms produce their own waste that contains harmful chemicals—these are absorbed back into our bodies, causing other problems.

The following chart shows the organic acid urine test result of a patient with toxic bacteria and yeast overgrowth in their intestines. The high levels of organic acids demonstrate that these bacteria make toxic chemicals that are absorbed into the blood, processed by the liver, and then excreted through the kidneys. This is an example of the body being poisoned internally by abnormal microbes in the gut, which is often a consequence of antibiotic use: good bacteria are killed off, and resistive, toxic bacteria and yeasts overgrow and survive.

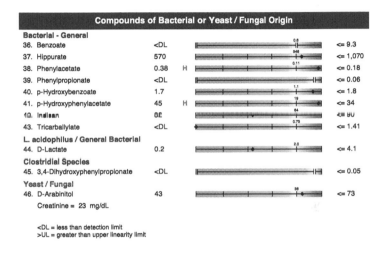

Compounds of Bacterial or Yeast / Fungal Origin		
Bacterial - General		
36. Benzoate	<DL	<= 9.3
37. Hippurate	570	<= 1,070
38. Phenylacetate	0.38 H	<= 0.18
39. Phenylpropionate	<DL	<= 0.06
40. p-Hydroxybenzoate	1.7	<= 1.8
41. p-Hydroxyphenylacetate	45 H	<= 34
42. Indican	0£	<= 90
43. Tricarballylate	<DL	<= 1.41
L. acidophilus / General Bacterial		
44. D-Lactate	0.2	<= 4.1
Clostridial Species		
45. 3,4-Dihydroxyphenylpropionate	<DL	<= 0.05
Yeast / Fungal		
46. D-Arabinitol	43	<= 73
Creatinine = 23 mg/dL		

<DL = less than detection limit
>UL = greater than upper linearity limit

THE CAUSES OF SMALL INTESTINE PROTEIN MALDIGESTION AND MALABSORPTION

Food sensitivity, intolerances, prescription medication, and unclean food (chemically saturated food), herbicides. SIBO, and toxic colonic bacteria, and yeast can damage the intestine's delicate membrane lining, which can cause secondary malabsorption of partially digested proteins.

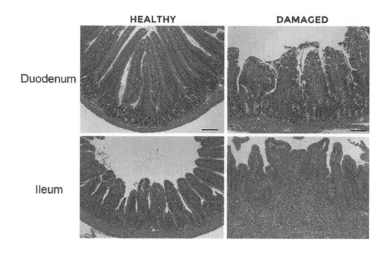

Once the partially digested proteins reach the small intestine, they undergo further breakdown by pancreatic enzymes and the enzymes in the villi of the small intestine.

The process of protein digestion is very complex, and if there are blocks at any point along the way, digestion may not occur. This leaves a person with inadequate amounts of essential amino acids to build or repair the body.

Additionally, all of the enzymes needed for the job are, of course, proteins, and one can get into the catch-22 that I mentioned earlier: They won't digest or absorb enough amino acids, and then won't have enough to even manufacture the enzymes *to do the digesting*. This happens more often than you think—it's not a rare occurrence. Refer to the chart for enzymes and their specific actions.

Proteolytic Enzymes and Their Actions

Secreted in	Enzymes Secreted	Action
Stomach	Pepsin	Converts complex proteins to small peptides
Pancreas	Trypsin	Specifically acts on peptide bonds contributed by basic amino acids like arginine, lysine & histidine
		Activates trypsinogen to trypsin
		Procarboxypeptidase to carboxypeptidase, Proelastase to elastase, and proaminopeptidase to aminopeptidase
	Chymotrypsin	Specifically acts on peptide bonds contributed by aromatic amino acids like phenylalanine, tyrosine, tryptophan
	Carboxypeptidase	Carboxy terminal amino acids
	Elastase	
Small Intestine	Amino Peptidase	Amino terminal amino acids
	Dipeptidase	Acts on dipeptides and releases free amino acids

In our clinic, we routinely measure levels of amino acids in the blood. This indicates whether or not a patient's diet and digestion result in normal blood amino acid levels. The following chart is the typical lab result we see from people who don't eat enough proteins, don't properly digest and absorb them. The levels of most of the essential amino acids are very low, which underlies many common health problems.

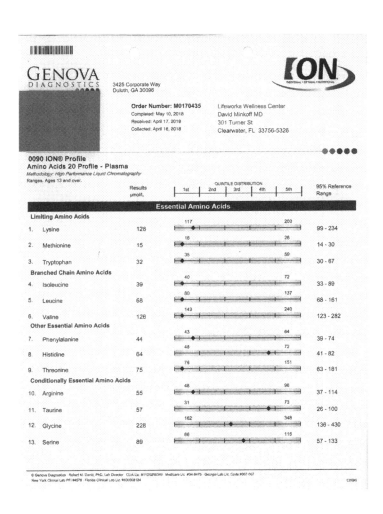

THE ROLE OF PERFECT AMINO

To solve these problems, you must handle the glitches along the way. One of the ways we bypass many of the barriers to digestion is by giving the patient Perfect Amino—the amino acids are already in a digested form, so we don't have to worry about the body taking care of this process.

In the formulation of supplemental amino acids, they come together with an L and R orientation, but the body can't use the right—the left form fits the structure, and the right simply doesn't fit. It's like putting a right-handed person in a row of left-handed people who are all trying to write a paper: the right-handed person will bump someone's arm because they don't fit the form.

Furthermore, since amino acids come in two forms: an L form, which is left; and an R form, which is right, many companies sell amino acids which are 50:50 of each. However, in human biology, only the L form can be used. Perfect Amino is ideal because it contains only the L form, and is of pharmaceutical-grade purity. Taken on an empty stomach with a glass of water or a sports drink, the amino acids are in the bloodstream within twenty-three minutes, even if you have impaired digestion in the stomach or small intestine.

Taking Perfect Amino is a powerful way to bypass the major system barriers our bodies have acquired due to our lifestyles and the plethora of drugs available today, prescribed or otherwise. When proteins are properly digested and absorbed, single amino acids are taken in by the small intestinal cells, put into the bloodstream, and sent to the cells of the body. Once they are there, they are reassembled into body proteins.

HOW PROTEINS ARE MADE

There is a wide range of complexity and amino acid combinations in body proteins. The most abundant proteins in the body are collagen (it's about 30 percent of all the proteins, which makes up the framework of the body), hemoglobin (the protein in red blood cells that carries oxygen and carbon dioxide), and muscle tissue. Among the estimated 20-50,000 other proteins are growth hormone, insulin, neurotransmitters, and many different enzymes.

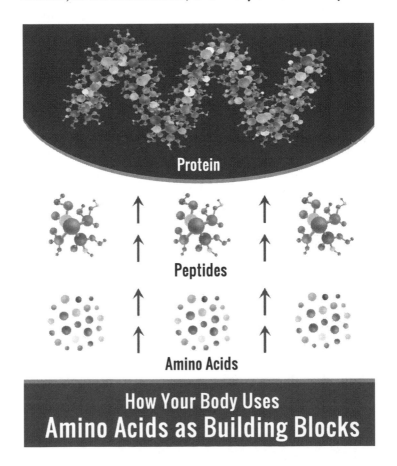

Protein

Peptides

Amino Acids

How Your Body Uses Amino Acids as Building Blocks

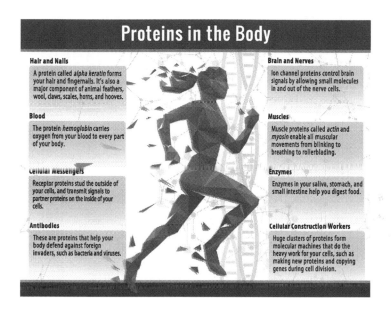

Proteins in the Body

Hair and Nails

A protein called *alpha keratin* forms your hair and fingernails. It's also a major component of animal feathers, wool, claws, scales, horns, and hooves.

Blood

The protein *hemoglobin* carries oxygen from your blood to every part of your body.

Cellular Messengers

Receptor proteins stud the outside of your cells, and transmit signals to partner proteins on the inside of your cells.

Antibodies

These are proteins that help your body defend against foreign invaders, such as bacteria and viruses.

Brain and Nerves

Ion channel proteins control brain signals by allowing small molecules in and out of the nerve cells.

Muscles

Muscle proteins called *actin* and *myosin* enable all muscular movements from blinking to breathing to rollerblading.

Enzymes

Enzymes in your saliva, stomach, and small intestine help you digest food.

Cellular Construction Workers

Huge clusters of proteins form molecular machines that do the heavy work for your cells, such as making new proteins and copying genes during cell division.

THE IMPORTANCE OF ENZYMES

Enzymes are required for digestion. They are the proteins that catalyze chemical reactions in a cell, and it's likely they were the first proteins synthesized in the ocean before biological life even existed. During the first few billion years of the earth's formation, there was ample nitrogen gas in the atmosphere, but very little oxygen; somehow, the nitrogen was incorporated into mixtures of carbon, hydrogen, and oxygen and the first amino acids were formed. Then, these amino acids combined into proteins that acted as facilitators for chemical reactions to occur more easily. These proteins are known as *enzymes*.

To illustrate how enzymes work, imagine that a muscle

cell has to manufacture more fibers. There are amino acids strewn all over the place within the cell. Now, the size of an amino acid in relation to the cell is like a piece of dust on planet earth—it's tiny. Suppose you want to manufacture the muscle protein *actin* that contains 6100 amino acids in its chain. How are you going to get all of those amino acids lined up in the right order—and they have to be *exactly* right—so the structure is perfect?

Think of it this way: amino acids float all over the place, and you need to get them into a specific order. The enzyme acts like a docking station (a slot that each amino acid can fall into), and they must fall into them in the right sequence, so they can bond. Now as enzymes are proteins, they have to be made in the same way! Only God knows how this ever got worked out. To make a protein, you have to get one amino acid next to another, and then next to another. They won't line up automatically if they just float around in the big space of a cell. The enzyme docking station provides a magnetic or chemical attraction so they move together and bond, and then manufacture a protein.

THE OTHER ROLE OF ENZYMES

Enzymes don't just build—they can also take things apart. Digestive enzymes can cleave bonds between amino acids. Since all processes that relate to manufacturing and modifying require energy, enzymes also burn the fuel of a cell and capture the energy released when it occurs. They also play a key role in detoxifying the body of poisonous waste matter and chemicals.

If you recall from Chapter One, enzymes from the pancreas like trypsin and chymotrypsin are able to pull apart long protein chains from milk, meat, beans, and nuts into individual amino acids—if you're already lacking in protein or essential amino acids, you can also have low digestive enzyme levels. We can measure a patient's chymotrypsin levels by testing their stool to see if they are making enough of it to digest food. We've found that many people age thirty-five and older have low chymotrypsin levels, most likely due to a lack of dietary essential amino acids.

When this is the case, the individual is stuck in a vicious cycle: Proteins arrive at the small intestine, but there is a lack of chymotrypsin to digest them; they don't absorb enough amino acids to make more chymotrypsin, and unfortunately, the cycle continues.

MEDIA'S INFLUENCE ON OUR HEALTH

Heartburn commercials are no strangers in the world of television advertising. The makers of Pepcid confidently tell us we can eat a hoagie with sausage and peppers and not feel any heartburn. It's the wrong message, and it indoctrinates the public so heavily that they believe the answer to their problem is another drug. "I'll just take this, and I'll be fine." Food allergies or intolerances can actually be the root cause of reflux for some people, but they think the solution is found in a pill. There is hard evidence that taking stomach acid blocking drugs are linked to higher early death risk and increases risks for cancer and other debilitative diseases.[10] Taking heartburn medication on a regular basis is comparable to numbing your hand with an anesthetic and then putting your hand on a hot stove. You won't feel the pain, but you'll smell the burning flesh, and you know that it isn't good for you. But since it doesn't hurt, you don't remove your hand.

Another large trend in the medical industry is the release of new antibiotic drugs to treat SIBO, but the drugs kill off all of the beneficial organisms—the person is often left in a worse state than before they started taking the drug! The three-drug combination for the bacterial infection *H Pylori* can produce the same result, and this puts patients at risk for potentially deadly bacteria, like C. Diff. However, when there's good acid in the stomach, these bacteria cannot live either. If modern medicine appreciated the intelligent design of the human body and worked *with* it to restore its natural functionality, most

---

10 Science News, "Popular heartburn drugs linked to higher early death risk," Science Daily, July 5, 2017, https://www.sciencedaily.com/releases/2017/07/170705113546.htm

of the health care being administered in the U.S. would be unnecessary.

I pity the poor people who go to the doctor because of heartburn or an ulcer—let's hope the gastroenterologist doesn't find *H. pylori* on an endoscopy. The patient will be prescribed a month or two of three different antibiotics that not only kill the bad bacteria, but also kill the good, natural flora in the intestine. Not only that, they will also breed overgrowth of yeasts and toxic bacteria that are *not* antibiotic-sensitive. It's unfortunate that people get into endless cycles and distort their normal physiology due to incorrect interventions, when there are better ways to restore normal function that won't lead to these issues.

Simple actions like restoring stomach acid with supplemental hydrochloric acid, adding pancreatic digestive enzymes, using probiotics to restore normal flora, and taking Perfect Amino to give the body the essential amino acids blend into a scenario that restores health—without the use of compromising drug therapies. These interventions usually work, and they are always worth a try if the practitioner is up to snuff.

THE SMALL INTESTINAL BARRIER AND LEAKY GUT

In most people, the small intestine is about twenty-five feet long, folded over itself numerous times. If you unfolded it, closed one end, and pumped air in, its surface area would be about the same as that of two tennis courts. Despite its huge area, it's very compact, and every little fold has another fold; there are villi and microvilli to maximize the area and absorb nutrients, and there are enzymes on the surface to aid in digestion activation.

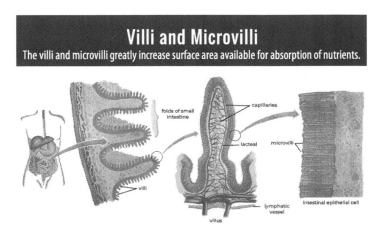

Villi and Microvilli
The villi and microvilli greatly increase surface area available for absorption of nutrients.

The inner lining of the small intestine is only one cell layer thick. In addition to the villi, there is a "glue" that holds these cells together. Let's say someone eats a steak and it enters the body as the big, long chain of about 6100 amino acids per fiber. The pepsin in the stomach will cut them down to five hundred amino acid chains. When the partially digested proteins reach the small intestine, the pancreatic enzymes cut them down to single amino acids, or into short chains of a few amino acids. If the chains are longer than that, they will not be absorbed by the microvilli—they will be too big.

If the tight junctions between the small intestinal cells are too permeable due to local injury (see the chart for causes), the longer chains can pass through the tight junctions into the bloodstream—this is known as leaky gut. It's "leaky" because substances that should never be allowed to enter the body do so through a "leak" in the intestinal wall barrier. The junction that was once tight is now open.

Our immune system considers most of these substances to be "foreign"—these are proteins that come from cows, pigs, bacteria, or parasites. As a safeguard, nature put three-fourths of our immune system within the wall of our small intestine as a shield against such invasions. This is known as the Gut Associated Lymphoid Tissue (GALT). When these foreign proteins pass through, an immune response is generated to target these invaders, and this process underlies most autoimmune diseases, like

Rheumatoid Arthritis and Lupus. The immune system becomes so agitated from the load of foreign proteins that it begins to attack similar proteins in its own body, thus the autoimmune reaction. The system turns against its own tissue, and much like what happens in a war with friendly fire, an airplane drops a bomb on its own troops by mistake.

Gastrointestinal Wall
Transection of the Small Intestine

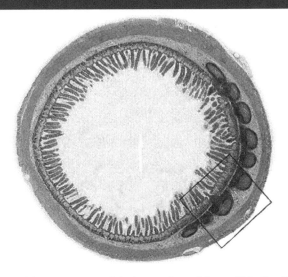

60 percent of the immune system is in the outer layer of the small intestine. This is known as the gut associated lymphoid tissue (GALT). This is our first layer of immune protection from microbes that can come across the intestinal wall with "leaky gut."

The protein that modulates the permeability of the tight junctions between the cells is called *zonulin*. If there is injury to the tight junction, the level of zonulin in the stool and bloodstream can increase and is considered to be an indicator of leaky gut. When the tight junctions are open, then bacteria and parasites can come across, also—these can be commonly identified in blood samples if they are viewed with certain microscopes. Please refer to the graphic.

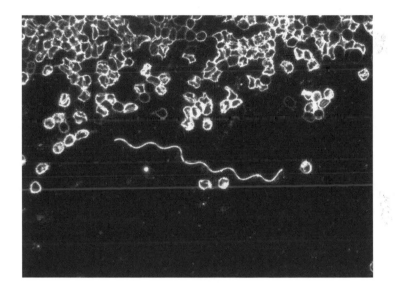

If there has been a great deal of damage to the small intestine due to drugs, bacteria, infection, and the like, the leak can be large and many foreign proteins can enter. The immune system then goes into a state of hyper action and hypervigilance—it sees "infidels" climbing over the wall, and it shoots anything that moves. This can result in severe, inflammatory autoimmune diseases, such as rheumatoid arthritis, lupus, and even multiple sclerosis.

Development of Leaky Gut
And Top Causes of Increased Zonulin

1) Low stomach acid and/or antibiotic therapy (These can cause the overgrowth of harmful organisms like yeast and SIBO)

2) Foods that contain gluten

3) Glyphosate pesticide residue on foods (For more information check out this link: https://www.Jillcarnahan.com/2013/07/14/Zonulin-Leaky-Gut/)

4) Virtually all pharmaceutical medications

5) Excess alcohol consumption

6) Nightshade vegetables or dairy proteins (in sensitive individuals)

THE MODERN-DAY EPIDEMIC OF AUTO-IMMUNE DISEASE

The unfortunate side effect of leaky gut is that we now have an epidemic of autoimmune disease—our immune system creates antibodies, mostly due to leaky gut and invading foreign particles. As proteins, cow muscle and cartilage look a lot like human protein, and since the foreign proteins resemble our own, the system begins to attack its own joints and cell nuclei.

We see autoimmune disease in the form of rheumatoid

arthritis, where the immune system attacks joints, or in lupus, where it attacks cell nuclei; or in multiple sclerosis, where it attacks *myelin*, the coating around nerve cells.

We see patient after patient at the clinic with these diseases, and through detailed testing, we discover that they have high amounts of environmental toxins, such as glyphosate, in their bodies. We also find that they have low levels of stomach acid, have yeast and parasites in their small intestine; a lack of normal bacterial flora in their colons; low levels of digestive enzymes from their pancreas; and low levels of amino acids in their blood. When we document these toxicities, infections, and deficiencies, we can begin the process to properly repair their physiology and restore their health without the use of drugs. Their leaky gut will seal, the auto-immune process ceases, and the disease will abate.

We've discussed the barriers to protein digestion and ways to overcome them, but not everyone will seek out these natural remedies. Since poor protein digestion leads to deficiency and this is still a common issue, we'll move into talking about the consequences to the body if this problem is allowed to continue.

CASE STUDY

One of our patients was a sixty-three-year-old female who'd had rheumatoid arthritis for ten years. The pain and swelling in her joints had been getting worse before she came to us. Her previous doctor put her on three strong anti-inflammatory drugs: plaquenil, prednisone, and methyltrexate. These were supposed to block her immune system so it could no longer attack her body, but they were not working. The doctor was prepared to put her on the "ultimate" new drug, Embril—one that carried grave warnings about causing cancer or tuberculosis (TB). The drug claimed to be effective, but it was dangerous.

The patient was afraid to take this drug, so she asked for our help. We did a stool test and discovered that she had two parasites, did not have enough good bacteria, and that her system was heavily colonized with yeast overgrowth. She also had severe deficiencies in amino acids, minerals, vitamins, and essential fatty acids. Once we identified her systemic issues, we targeted them so her body could heal. We began a program to restore her intestinal flora, kill the pathogens with natural herbal remedies, and rehabilitate the integrity of her intestinal membrane—she took a lot of Perfect Amino, along with many other supplements and intravenous fluids. Within five months, her joint pain was gone and the swelling had lessened considerably. She felt really good and said she "felt like a new gal."

Before she started our treatment program, she had been tested by her rheumatologist due to the worsening of her condition. Her initial tests were positive for antinuclear antibody (ANA), rheumatoid factor, and an elevated sedimentation rate (which was an indicator of inflammation in the body). We retested her after she had followed our recommended protocols, and her antinuclear antibody and rheumatoid factor had both gone negative. Her sedimentation rate also dropped from sixty to a normal reading of fifteen.

During our treatment process, she was able to wean off the prednisone and methyltrexate. She asked me if she had to go back to the rheumatologist, and I told her that she didn't—handling her disease process our way had worked very well, and she should continue to remain healthy in the future. "But," I added, "If you could go back just one more time, for me, and show him your results, I'd appreciate it. If he asks what you've done to see these improvements, show him your lab work and tell him you went to the natural doctor. If he needs assistance with any of his other patients, I'd be happy to help."

CHAPTER FIVE

CONSEQUENCES OF PROTEIN DEFICIENCY

We've established that inadequate protein intake can cause devastating results. A lack of nutrition along with environmental toxicity are the reasons for the poor health we experience today. Never before in human history has the human race suffered from epidemics like diabetes, Alzheimer's Disease, Parkinson's, ALS, osteoporosis, obesity, cancers, Lyme disease, chronic fatigue, and countless other problems.

We've also established that an inability to digest enough protein contributes to the increase in health issues and disease. Patients come into the clinic and we discover they haven't been eating or digesting well; they're toxic because they're unaware of what they've been putting into their bodies, or what they've been exposed to.

We examine them and then help reverse harmful processes to get them back to a healthier state—to put the brakes on their body's downhill slide and help it climb back up, we need to reduce their toxic load. This always involves rebuilding their protein nutrition along with the rest of their nutritional needs like vitamin, mineral, and essential fatty acid intake.

Patients with inadequate protein might also be unable to detoxify. The urine test we run identifies twenty-four different categories of environmental toxins; if there are high levels of any of them, we know the body isn't getting rid of them efficiently, or the person is being poisoned without realizing it. We discover toxins like gasoline additives, Styrofoam, plastics, fumigants, pesticides, and dry-cleaning fluids, to name a few.

Interestingly enough, if we test two people who live in the same house, these toxins can appear in one person's urine and not the other. For example, a wife's detoxification pathways might work well because she has an adequate intake of amino acids and minerals. Her husband, on the other hand, might have a low level of amino acids—making him unable to create enzymes to detoxify—and this makes him sick. Some of the ability to detoxify is genetic, but much of it is related to the person's health and nutrition.

THE TOXIC GIRL

A twelve-year-old girl in Florida gradually became tired and lethargic—she had trouble doing her homework, and she complained that she could not "think," do her math problems, or write her essays. She just wanted to lie in bed and rest. After nine months, there had been no change in her condition. She was seen by twenty different doctors in various locations including the Pediatric University Hospital. They concluded that she had a psychiatric problem, so they put her on psychiatric medications, but they did not help.

Eventually, her parents brought her in to see me, and I ran a panel for environmental toxins. All of the tests came back negative except for one that revealed extremely high levels of the gasoline octane booster additives HTBE and MTBE in her system. Virtually everyone on the planet has some level of these additives in their system because gasoline fumes are everywhere, and by inhalation, they enter our bodies. Per the lab, normal measurements of these additives are under two hundred, but they are considered acceptable up to eight-hundred. However, this girl's level was 39,000! The lab was very concerned when they called to tell me, as this was the highest level they'd ever seen in a child. I asked the parents if the girl was sniffing gasoline, washing her hands in it, or taking cars apart. A light dawned on them and they said, "Oh, my goodness! A couple of years ago she decided that she wanted to be the next Danica Patrick and win a NASCAR race; she's been taking driving lessons in midget race cars on the weekends for the past couple of years."

We discovered that the girl had been inhaling gas fumes from race car exhaust, and that she couldn't detoxify effectively. She also had a leaky gut and amino acid deficiencies. When we got her to detoxify her body of the chemicals, her brain turned "back on." This goes to show that we need to consider toxins and other harmful substances in the body as the sources of illness and disease. If we fail to do so, there's no way for doctors, patients, or parents to identify or eliminate them as possible causes if and when sickness occurs.

This girl's case was extreme, but it's not uncommon for us to find toxins present in a patient's system. I do case after case of amino acid testing, comparing the eight essential amino levels in each person; I'll find one that's really low and then another. A typical scenario might be discovering that a person has a bad gut with five bacteria that shouldn't be there, as well as three parasites. They can't detoxify, and their health will continue to decline if they don't begin treatment.

OTHER CONSEQUENCES

It's a relatively well-known fact that between the ages of

twenty and sixty, the average person loses a significant amount of lean body mass, bone strength, muscle, and organ tissue. We usually chalk this up to aging, but this is certainly not always the case. For most people, the gradual loss of lean body mass is due to a lack of stimulus and inadequate absorption of amino acids.

For example, I have a seventy-six-year-old friend who is still a bodybuilder. He works out five hours a day to keep his physique and he's built like the Hulk, with only three percent body fat. Given the right genes, nutrition, and workout ethic, aging bodies can keep their fitness and muscle mass.

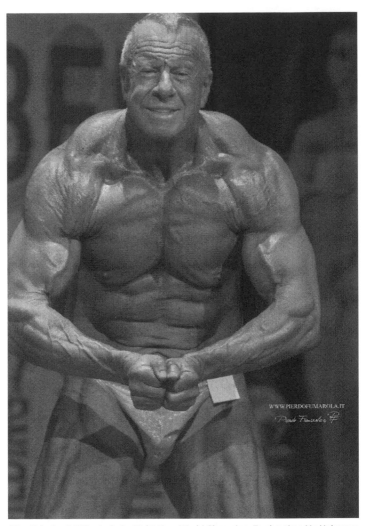

WWW.PIERDOFUMAROLA.IT

Dion Friedland. Titles include: Eight-time World Champion; Twelve-time Mr. Universe; Twelve-time Mr. Europe; Five-time Serge Nubret Champion; IFBB Grand Prix de France Open Champion; IBFF Mr. International Champion; and Four-time Mr. Galaxy Champion.

Adequate nutrition can maintain lean body mass or at least slow its reduction with aging. Older adults can still manufacture proteins if given the right ingredients—getting older doesn't mean you have to dwindle away. If you keep up the exercise stimulus and your nutrition is good, you can maintain lean body mass while aging.

REBUILDING IN YOUR GOLDEN YEARS

I gave the example of my body building friend, and you might think that he naturally maintains lean body mass due to his active lifestyle. But what about a sixty-five-year-old who has been inactive for a long time, and has lost a significant amount of muscle mass? Can they rebuild? It's difficult to measure, but most people are able to regain a worthwhile amount of mass. Of course, in some cases, the mass may be too far gone and there's not much that can be done, but overall, it's possible to turn it around. Women with osteoporosis, for example, can rebuild their bone structure by increasing their intake of vitamin D, amino acids, and hormones. However, they can't rely completely on medicine; they have to squat and lift other weights to provide the proper stimulus. The bottom line is, it's never too late to start again! In fact, sometimes older people get the most response from these positive changes, because they have the most room for improvement.

CASE STUDY

A doctor made this type of improvement apparent at a long-term-care home in Hawaii. The residents were elderly people who couldn't take care of themselves anymore; many had Alzheimer's or simply had no strength. When this doctor gave them essential amino acids and nutritious food with vitamins, minerals, and enzymes, he found that many times, within a few months of taking them, patients began to function at higher levels—they could get out of bed, dress themselves, and walk down the hall. Their thinking processes also improved: people who formerly could not find their way to the cafeteria had no trouble getting there, and those who used to just sit in a chair all interacted socially with others. This doctor provided other nutrition in addition to the amino acids, but they played a large role in the tremendous improvement of the patients.

So far, we've discussed my research experience and how I've treated patients with various health issues. I've discovered that amino acid supplementation addresses the protein problem while simultaneously alleviating digestive complications. In the next section of the book, we'll discuss how the protein problem affects different subgroups of people.

PART TWO

SPECIFIC PROBLEMS FOR SUB-GROUPS

CHAPTER SIX

SPECIFIC TO WOMEN

While most protein products are marketed toward men and bodybuilding, the protein problem affects women in many specific ways. These include osteoporosis, hormone deficiency, beauty concerns such as sagging skin and wrinkles, loss of muscle mass, and problems during menopause.

PROTEIN'S CONNECTION TO OSTEOPOROSIS IN WOMEN

If you believe what commercials say on TV, taking calcium is the solution to osteoporosis—just take it and you'll be fine. If that doesn't work, they suggest taking a bisphosphonate drug. This medication will make your bones look better on a density scan, but in reality, it makes them very fragile. In some cases, the drug even causes a condition called osteonecrosis, in which bone cells die, and the jaw bone disintegrates. Other minor side effects like joint and muscle pain, nausea, heartburn and ulcers have also been reported. A good review of the efficacy of bisphosphonates concludes that there are no proven clinical benefits in postmenopausal women.[11] Due to the small potential of benefit and high risk, I do not consider them a worthwhile treatment option.

While increasing calcium intake can be beneficial, if one has a calcium-deficient diet, it's important to understand that demineralized bone is rubbery like old celery—minerals only stick if a protein matrix is present. Bones are constructed like a 1950s lath and plaster wall; thin lath strips were nailed horizontally across wall studs, and then plaster was spread over them. The lath gave the plaster something to stick to, and created the wall interior. In a similar fashion, bones need a dense matrix of protein as a structural foundation before "overlaying" the calcium. This foundation is collagen, the most abundant structural protein in the body.

Roughly 50 percent of bone by weight is collagen, which is a protein, and osteoporosis occurs when there is a loss of collagen. By rebuilding it, you can rebuild bones. Collagen

---

11   Therapeutics Letter, "A Systematic Review of the Efficacy of Bisphosphonates," Therapeutics Initiative, January 24, 2012, https://www.ti.ubc.ca/2012/01/24/a-systematic-review-of-the-efficacy-of-%EF%BF%BC%EF%BF%BCbisphosphonates/

is made of amino acids and other essential components so that the mineral content of bone—mainly calcium and phosphorous—has something to attach to. Other critical elements needed to build bone are: vitamin D, vitamin K, and hormones (thyroid, estrogen, progesterone, DHEA and testosterone). Vitamin B6 and magnesium are also important for proper collagen formation.

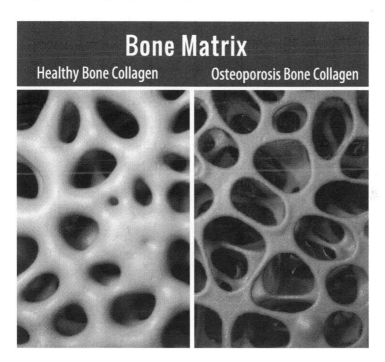

Bone Matrix

Healthy Bone Collagen · Osteoporosis Bone Collagen

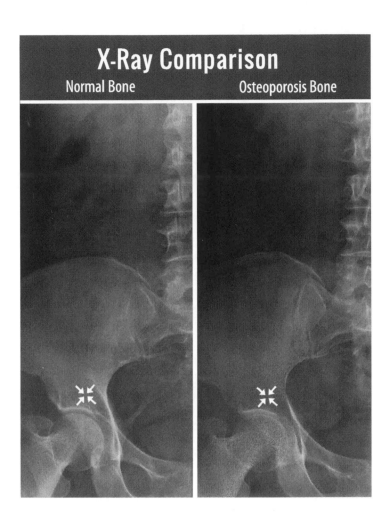

X-Ray Comparison

Normal Bone | Osteoporosis Bone

The other important factor in building bones is targeted exercise—the bones must undergo enough stress to stay strong. Experiments using two simple exercises, deadlifts and squats, have shown great results if coupled with the nutritional advice listed above. With proper instruction from a trained exercise coach or instructor, do three sets of ten repetitions of deadlifts and squats, twice per week to see results. These movements can be done with no weights to start, but as the person gets stronger, weights should be added. This type of resistance training is extremely effective at building bone. In our clinic we have patients do the exercises on a power plate, their bone density improves at an even faster rate. The power plate was developed by NASA for astronauts because while they are in space with no gravity, they are prone to get osteoporosis. By giving their bodies a vibratory stimulus, it encourages their bodies to keep their bone.

CASE STUDY

We often find low serum amino acid levels in women with osteoporosis. When we give these women extra doses of amino acids and treat other factors within their systems that may not be in good shape, their bones re-mineralize. This was the case with Betty, age sixty-eight.

Betty came into the clinic after her regular doctor checked her bone density and confirmed that it was in the osteoporosis range. He told her that she needed to greatly increase her calcium intake, and to begin taking Fosomax (bisphosphonate) medication. She had read reports of the medication's potential side effects and was seeking another opinion.

After seeing her and running laboratory tests we found the usual deficiencies that we see in this situation: low red blood cell magnesium and selenium, very low vitamin D and iodine, low pancreatic chymotrypsin for protein digestion, low serum essential amino acids, low progesterone and testosterone, bacterial overgrowth in her small intestine with a roundworm parasite, and nearly absent stomach acid. She also had very low levels of estrogen, testosterone, DHEA, and progesterone. We started a program to address her nutritional and hormonal deficiencies, and to improve her gut, digestion, and absorption. We also began the weight training program described above with a power plate, three times per week. A recheck of her bone density in six months showed vast improvement, and after a year and a half, she was back in the normal range for her age.

This case study shows us that these problems are reversible, and treatment can be administered by a knowledgeable nutritional practitioner. A good doctor knows what to find and fix, and then the body will take over—inherently, it knows what to do. This is health restoration at its best.

PROTEIN'S CONNECTION TO LOW THYROID IN WOMEN

It is estimated that at least 60 percent of the U.S. population is thyroid hormone deficient. This includes both men and women. Unfortunately, many people go undiagnosed because the current medical standard does not accurately reflect what "normal" really is. If a patient goes to a doctor and says, "I'm gaining weight, I'm tired, my hair is thinning, my skin is dry, and I'm a little constipated—something is wrong." The doctor and patient often assume something is going on with the thyroid, and the doctor will run a test called TSH to check for their level of thyroid stimulating hormone. The normal range for most labs is 0.5 to 4.5, and if the patient is within this range, most doctors will consider that the patient is fine and chalk the symptoms up to something else. Disgruntled patients come to my practice and tell me that they were told they are tired because they are getting older, they're depressed, or it's just the change of life setting in. Many will stop looking for solutions and just accept it because their doctor "told them so, and of course, he knows best."

DO REFERENCE RANGES DEFINE NORMALITY?

There's a bell curve when it comes to determining the thyroid hormone levels of patients. The "normal levels" do not come from a population that is screened for health—feeble eighty-year-olds with cancer and seventeen-year-old top athletes are included in the "normal" range. So, this test is not an accurate reflection of what the optimum thyroid level should be in a patient.

According to the ZRT Laboratory blog: The real question that needs to be answered is: where does the "normal" standard come from? Reference ranges do not always reflect a normal healthy population with bodies that are free of medications. Most laboratories establish their reference ranges based on a large population of people where detailed information on health status, stage of life (premenopausal vs. postmenopausal), hormone levels, and medications used is unknown. Therefore, those factors are not taken into account. Couple this with differences in lifestyles, physiology, dietary habits, and genetic heredity, and it's even more difficult to define—let alone find—a normal population.[12]

When we measure tyrosine and iodine levels in the blood of thyroid patients, we often discover that both are also low. (Tyrosine is an amino acid that the body makes into thyroid hormone when it is combined with iodine.) When these levels are low, we work to rebuild their tyrosine and iodine levels. Some patients may need thyroid hormone in the meantime, but in quite a few cases, once their levels

---

12   Groves, Margaret, "How Reference Ranges Determine a 'Normal' Lab Test Result," The ZRT Laboratory Blog, November 13, 2015, http://blog.zrtlab.com/reference-ranges

of tyrosine and iodine are back to normal, along with their magnesium, selenium, and vitamin C, their body starts to make thyroid hormone on its own again. When the patient was deficient in these critical nutrients, the thyroid could not produce what was required. However, once they were present, normal function was restored, and they could then wean off prescription thyroid therapy.

IS IT LOW THYROID?

When I schedule a talk at the local library or health food store with the title "I Saw My Doctor Because I Think I Have Low Thyroid, But He Won't Treat Me Because My TSH is Normal," we get a standing-room-only crowd. After the talk, people realize that they most likely *do* have low thyroid, and need to seek out a nutritionally-oriented MD who can measure all of the thyroid hormones, determine the optimum levels for them as an individual, and administer the correct treatment. People are relieved when they finally get their thyroid hormone to its ideal levels for their body—they are no longer feeling sluggish, cold, gaining weight, or stuck in a pattern of foggy, slow thinking. For years, their best authority, their doctor, told them they were fine, when in fact, they were not. When they finally discover the answer, patients are ecstatic, but they're also angry. And rightly so!

CASE STUDY

Jennifer came to us after seeing her family practitioner because she kept gaining weight. She was also having trouble getting through her day at work. "I'm just so tired at the end of the day. I can hardly function. I saw my doctor and I told him that low thyroid runs in my family; both my sister and mother are on therapy. He ordered a TSH (thyroid stimulating hormone test). He told me the regular normal levels were 0.5–4.5, and mine came back 4.4. He said he could not prescribe me thyroid medication because I was in the normal range. I pleaded with him, but he said if the Board of Medicine ever found out, he might get in trouble. In my frustration, I started looking around and I found you."

We tested her, and sure enough her TSH was 4.4, but her Free T3 (the active hormone) was 2.1, with the normal range being 2-4.5. Her Free T4 was 0.9, with normal being 0.9-4.5. She was clearly on the very low end of "normal" values. I started her on prescription Naturethroid medicine, which contains animal thyroid gland and the active hormones that she needed.

We gradually increased her dose until her hands and body were nice and warm, she had no cold sensitivity, and she had better energy with no afternoon lull. After a couple of months, she resumed exercising and lost eight pounds. During initial testing, we discovered that she had low tyrosine and iodine, so we also put her on supplemental amino acids (Perfect Amino) and iodine in addition to the Naturethroid. Repeat blood testing revealed normal levels of TSH, Free T3, Free T4, tyrosine and iodine. She was grateful and happy for the positive changes, but after six months she called because she thought her thyroid levels might be too high!

She was feeling hyper, her heart rate had increased, and she was having trouble sleeping. I measured her thyroid blood levels and they were high, so I began to wean her off the prescription. Within two months, she was off the medication and her body had normalized. This doesn't always happen, but it goes to show that the body can often heal itself when given the right nutrition to do so.

PROTEIN'S CONNECTION TO BEAUTY CONCERNS IN WOMEN

Sagging skin, bone loss, and hair loss are all critical concerns of women related to the protein problem. There is a published study showing that over a month's period of time, feeding people two thousand calories per day of mainly vegetables and some fruits, and walking for an hour a day along with three servings per day of an essential amino acid blend identical to Perfect Amino, that they lost significant weight, but didn't have sagging skin under the chin or other areas of the body. The body burned up fat, but didn't pirate protein for calories.[13]

When we administered the human chorionic gonadotropin hormone (HCG) diet to a few hundred patients, they had similar results. (HCG is often used in weight loss treatments, and is now only available through injection). HCG is the hormone of pregnancy, but if used as a therapy along with a very low-fat and calorie-restricted diet, it can facilitate significant weight loss. To give an example, let's say a patient is allowed five hundred calories per day for twenty-one days, with almost no fat. They also receive an injection of one hundred twenty-five units of HCG every day. Most patients won't be hungry, and

---

13 Luca-Moretti M, Grandi A, Luca E, Muratori G, Nofroni MG, Mucci MP, Gambetta P, Stimolo R, Drago P. Guidice G, Tamburlin N, "Master amino acid Pattern as substitute for dietary proteins during a weight-loss diet to achieve the body's nitrogen balance equilibrium with essentially no calories," pubmed.gov, September-October 2003, https://www.ncbi.nlm.nih.gov/pubmed/14964348

they will lose anywhere from twelve to twenty pounds in that short period of time. This diet is very safe when administered under doctor supervision, and in patients with high blood pressure and high blood sugar, it almost always normalizes their values. This diet can be a "quick start" to reset their pituitary gland, and then they can go back to a more normal, healthy diet.

Normally, with calorie-restricted diets, for every four pounds of body weight lost, one pound is lean body mass—that is not healthy. We found that if we gave patients two doses of Perfect Amino every day during a low-calorie diet, they were able to preserve lean body mass, and the majority of the weight loss came from fat. This was a much healthier approach because they didn't lose the essential structure of their bodies.

MENOPAUSE

During menopause, falling levels of hormones cause many undesirable effects in a woman's body. The role of these hormones is to keep cells nurtured so women are hearty enough to become pregnant and carry a fetus to term. Thus, these hormones have a building effect and keep the body more youthful. With falling hormone levels, this effect is lost, and lean body tissue begins to break down. Loss of bone, skin collagen, muscle mass, brain cells, and neurotransmitters all lead to more rapid aging, and the feeling that one is getting old. Wrinkles, weakness, osteoporosis, sagging skin, and a loss of energy occurs—this is not something any woman looks forward to. However, if whole-body nutrition—especially with essential amino acids—is maintained, women can age more gracefully into their 90's and beyond!

For many women, the reality check of a daily look in the mirror can determine their entire outlook for the day. When they are able to think, "Gee, my skin has few wrinkles, my eyes are bright, my hair is thick and full, and I have some muscles over my shoulders," that creates an optimistic attitude to start the day. These are the desirable effects of good protein nutrition, and they can go a long way in aiding both physical health and a positive mental outlook.

My wife is postmenopausal, and when she misses taking Perfect Amino for even one day, she notices that she doesn't have as much energy. Through personal experience and all that I have seen with patients, I believe that having adequate essential amino acids in the diet allows the aging body to make the necessary enzymes for energy production, detoxification, neurotransmitters, and muscle building—it can help to greatly slow the aging process.

Increasing amino acid intake is helpful for women experiencing menopause, but is it also effective in treating the health concerns of younger women. Consider for a moment that a woman loses about a pint of blood during menstruation. Blood is largely protein, and during the next month, the body has to manufacture anew all the blood that was lost. It needs lots of essential amino acids to do this, along with iron and other nutrients.

Another issue is that premenstrual syndrome (PMS) can be intense for some women. Bloating, moodiness, lack of energy, and pain all are difficult to bear. In most of the women we see, these symptoms are associated with a lack of progesterone being produced in the second half of the cycle. The reason for this lack is not entirely understood, but the combination of nutritional deficiencies and environmental toxins certainly play a role. So, adequate intake of vitamins, minerals, essential fats, and essential amino acids can help restore normal hormone production.

CASE STUDY

Jill is a twenty-seven-year-old career gal. She is in charge of IT at a large company in our area. Her health had always been good, but her PMS was bad. Beginning about a week before her cycle she became moody, anxious, and very intolerant of anyone, including her husband and her mother. She was also losing hair and having problems sleeping. Her mother and husband accompanied her to her first visit, and honestly, they looked about as desperate as she was.

"I need help," she said. "If I can't get this under control, both my beloved mother and husband are going to leave me." She told me she had become a vegan a few years before, thinking it was going to be healthy for her. Through lab testing, we discovered that she had severe deficiencies of essential amino acids, low magnesium, very low progesterone, and multiple vitamin deficiencies. I asked her to change her diet to a Paleo-type eating program, so she added organic meats, fish, and eggs back into her diet, while keeping up a high intake of vegetables. We added digestive enzymes, Perfect Amino, and a whole supplement program; we also added a little OTC progesterone cream. I asked her to come back for a recheck in three months.

When she returned, she was bright and cheery. "Look at me! My hair and nails are growing so well—they look nice, and they glisten. In fact, I am having to see my stylist more often because of faster hair growth. And see my muscles? She smiled as she flexed her biceps. You really helped me! Oh, and most importantly, my PMS is not an issue anymore. My family and I are back in love. I don't know how they put up with me so long."

BEYOND HEALING

It doesn't matter if you're young or elderly, male or

female—keeping up protein nutrition is of paramount importance. You may want external markers of beauty such as nice hair, skin, and nails, or shapely muscles as markers of strength. Or you may want strong blood, immune proteins, hormones, or neurotransmitters as indicators of healthy internal biochemistry. Whatever your goal, all of those factors depend on keeping up your levels of essential amino acids, and maintaining the chain of oral intake, digestion, and absorption and cellular utilization. All health and healing depend on this, no matter your age.

CHAPTER SEVEN

SPECIFIC TO ATHLETES

Athletes come into the clinic with the goal of improving their health, athletic performance, or body composition. Since I'm an athlete myself, I enjoy helping them, and their results are always of great interest to me.

Athletes often face problems with injury and recovery. They'll say, "I'm getting injured more often. I don't seem to have enough energy to perform, and my recovery time is too long." Many of these athletes lack adequate amounts of amino acids, and their bodies can't keep up with the demand that is being put on them. When we add Perfect Amino to their programs, they notice a dramatic difference.

On any given day, I'll go on a hard five-mile-run, and then head to the ocean to swim another mile as fast as

I can. My neighbor, on the other hand, takes his dog for a leisurely twenty-minute walk, twice a day. There is a big difference between the level of wear and tear on my body versus his. He might get along fine with a couple of servings of protein each day, but that wouldn't be enough for me—active bodies require more nutrition.

Soreness is a concern for athletes and is caused by the muscles being broken down. When athletes get what they need, the recovery process begins immediately, and they won't be sore the next day, or even the day after. If amino acids are replaced quickly, their muscles will heal at a faster rate.

Sometimes, people train so hard that they overstress their system and don't benefit from it; instead, they go into a breakdown, experience a decrease in adrenaline and cortisol, and lose energy. They may be sore or tired for a few days, or have several nights of restless sleep, because they are lacking much-needed protein—this leads to diminished returns when training. With enough amino acids and other strategic nutrition, athletes can avoid the breakdown, become stronger, and maintain high performance—even when they put massive stress on the body. It's helpful for athletes to take their last dose of Perfect Amino before bed. Growth hormones spike during sleep, and that's when the body does the majority of its recovery and repair.

THE WALK ACROSS THE TAKLIMAKAN DESERT IN CHINA

In a study published in Advances in Therapy Volume 20/4 2003, a fifty-one-year-old female racewalker walked across the Taklimakan desert in China—a distance of three hundred-forty-two miles in twenty-four days. Weather conditions were extremely harsh while she walked, ranging from twenty-three to eighty-six degrees Fahrenheit during the day. The desert terrain consisted of sand dunes with a lot of ups and downs, and she carried a fifty-pound backpack as she crossed the desert alone. Her diet consisted of taking eight tablets of Perfect Amino three times per day, plus vitamins, minerals, and a blended drink of carbs and fats, for a total caloric intake of three-thousand per day.[14]

Before embarking on the journey, a variety of exercise tests, laboratory blood tests, and body composition tests were conducted; they were also repeated upon her completion of the walk. By using the essential amino acid blend contained in Perfect Amino, results showed that she: 1) increased muscle mass, strength, and endurance. Her initial heart rate walking at eight kilometers per hour was one hundred-forty-nine, and at finish it was

---

14   Luca-Moretti M, Grandi A, Luca E, Mariani E, Vender G, Arrigotti E, Ferrario M, Rovelli E, "Results of Taking Master Amino Acid Pattern as a Sole and Total Substitute of Dietary Proteins in an Athlete During a Desert Crossing," Advances in Therapy, Volume 20, No. 4, July/August 2003, https://naturalsolutions.nz/articles/MAP-as-dietary-protein-substitute-in-Athlete-Crossing-Desert-Aug2003.pdf

one hundred-twenty-eight; 2) decreased fat mass by 20 percent, and had improved cardiovascular performance with a 15 percent improvement in VO2 max; and 3) had increased red blood cells, hemoglobin, and hematocrit. The conclusion was that using the Perfect Amino formula as the sole substitute for dietary protein in conjunction with extreme physical exercise can optimize body protein synthesis, as well as improve performance.

PREPPING FOR THE TOUR

Earlier in the book I talked about my friend and patient who provided nutritional strategies for one of the American teams doing the Tour de France. The race always begins the first weekend of July, and one year in March, one of their riders developed a bad parasitic infection with lots of diarrhea and malabsorption. He became very weak and lost muscle mass. The medical staff strongly doubted he'd recover by July and be physically prepared for twenty-one, high-intensity days of grueling physical activity.

My friend consulted me about this problem, and we were able to figure out what the infection was. Since there was severe protein malnutrition, I suggested we put the rider on Perfect Amino. All were amazed that in just over three short months he was race ready, won a mountain tour stage on a breakaway, and had his best Tour ever! This recovery and result, along with the race walker's successful walk across the Taklimakan, proved to me that amino acid supplementation can create physiological improvements in athletes.

CASE STUDY

Cherie G is notably the best masters Ironman athlete of all time. She has won Age Group Hawaii Ironman World Championships an unprecedented thirteen times, and Ironman 70.3 World Championships three times. She has done this from age sixty to her current age of seventy-four and she is still winning. According to Cherie, her ability to continue to put in high training hours to compete in these grueling events is largely due to her use of Perfect Amino. They allow her to recover and train the next day. To find out more about Cherie, you can read her Foreword at the beginning of the book.

PROTEIN'S CONNECTION TO LACK OF ENDURANCE AND PERFORMANCE IN ATHLETES

Performance improvement begins at the cellular level—energy systems must be stressed and stimulated to produce more energy. Cells contain factory-like structures, called *mitochondria,* where oxygen is combined with fuel to make adenosine triphosphate (ATP), the molecule that stores cellular energy. When stressed, the cell manufactures more mitochondria per cell, so that it can produce more energy in the form of ATP—when you become more physically fit, the cells get "fitter" too!

The ability to manufacture more energy depends on the number of mitochondria per cell, but within the mitochondria there are enzymes that actually take the calories from our food and turn them into ATP. So as there are more mitochondria, there must be a great increase in energy pathway enzymes to facilitate this process.

Since the structure of mitochondria, enzymes, muscle fibers, and tendons is composed of protein, there is a great need for essential amino acids for this process to occur. If we have adequate essential amino acid intake, all of these systems can improve. If we don't, then working out may produce little or no gain, as the deficiency of essential amino acids will limit the result. If you are working out and seeing no improvement in muscle strength, speed, endurance, or power, then this may be at the heart of your problem. However, you also want to take into account the other important components of this growth cycle: thyroid hormone, growth hormone, and insulin.

A STORY OF ENDURANCE

Another world-class athlete I've worked with is a former professional triathlete and three-time Ironman World Champion. He is one of very few people to win this event more than twice, and he has competed seven or eight times. He always arrived in Kona three weeks early for final preparation and to gauge whether or not he was truly in "good shape."

Compared to the average athlete, Ironman competitors train forty hours a week and are indeed in shape. A sample training schedule might be twenty hours on the bike for two hundred and fifty to three hundred miles; eight hours of running for a total of fifty to sixty miles; and then swimming up to thirty thousand yards. Then, they'll throw in weight training and stretching for good measure. They end up having a six-to-eight-hour day of exercise training, which is a lot of stress on the body.

To prepare for this rigorous training, this athlete began taking ten grams of Perfect Amino, two to three times per day, three months before his third Ironman attempt. On one of his bike training days prior to the event, he completed the one hundred and forty-mile course *thirty minutes faster* than any of his previous times. He called me in a panic, thinking there must be some kind of drug in the product and, he'd be disqualified—I assured him it was a pure, World Anti-Doping Association (WADA) tested, certified product. He went on to win his third Ironman title and retired that year. Later, he attributed his incredible results to Perfect Amino.

PERFECT AMINO AND THE OLYMPICS

One of my clients is a chiropractor who works with world-class track and field athletes. They've earned a dozen medals in the last two summer Olympic games while incorporating Perfect Amino into their nutrition program. As a doctor, he knows the power of nutrition in the competitive athlete. "Without superior nutrition, nothing that we do in the weight room or on the track will work. We stress the body so it will improve, but it will only improve if it receives the nutritional components needed to meet the demands of training and heal. That is why amino acid nutrition is so important."

PERFECT AMINO IN THE WEIGHT ROOM

A Miami fitness boot camp instructor and elite weight-lifting coach previously instructed his athletes take two hundred grams of whey protein each day to help them bulk up; nearly every one of them ended up with GI side effects, like gas and bloating. I suggested he give them Perfect Amino instead of the whey—he made the switch, and his athletes loved it! They have seen performance improvement, and their stomachs have settled down as well.

ATHLETES AND SICKNESS

As I mentioned earlier in the book, the body has two main functions when it's under stress from exercise training: keep the immune system up and running and repair structures and tissues. These include muscles, tendons, ligaments, and enzymes. If there is a nutritional deficiency, the body has to choose between these two tasks. It's common for athletes to get sick a few days after hard training or completing a big race, because the body may choose to repair structural elements and neglect the needs of the immune system. This is especially true if they lack essential amino acids—if the immune system is not supported, a cold or infection can ensue.

Personally, I'm very careful about this. For example, I did a race recently, and I took extra doses of Perfect Amino for a few days leading up to the event, and then immediately after, for a few days until all the soreness was gone, and I had completely recovered. I ran hard and did well on a hot race day, and I didn't get sick afterward because I took the extra doses to keep my immunity up.

As an athlete, I love to put forth effort, push my body, and feel the sweat and the pump—I love to compete. The worst days are the ones when my body is overworked or I'm sick or injured—I have to mope around and wait until I bounce back. Using essential amino acids like Perfect Amino allows the body to stay in a high state of immune health and to recover and to perform well. For me, amino acid nutrition is the cornerstone of being able to compete at a high level.

CHAPTER EIGHT

SPECIFIC TO THE ELDERLY

It's not unexpected that the protein problem affects the elderly, and we address this at the clinic through an anti-aging practice. Many older people come to us and say, "My memory isn't great, and I don't have energy like I used to. Can you help me?" People don't want to feel or "act" old, and amino acid supplementation can help.

Part of the breakdown that is experienced in old age is often related to poor nutrition. Some of the elderly can't afford a high-nutrition diet, and some simply don't know what good nutrition looks like—they don't eat well or don't supplement correctly. Breakfast might be a bowl of Corn Flakes with a cup of coffee and that meal doesn't provide strength or fuel for the body. This lack of nutrition leads to the body becoming weak, and the person becomes symptomatic—they don't function as well as they used to. Part of this problem can be attributed to low amino acid levels, which leads to low levels of hormones, neurotransmitters, bone loss, and loss of muscle strength.

The protein synthesis with Perfect Amino is *fast,* and there can be an immediate systematic difference. For example, we've done work with elderly people who had lost strength and couldn't get up from a chair without difficulty. We gave them ten grams of Perfect Amino, waited about forty-five minutes, and they were able to stand more easily.

THE CONNECTION TO ALZHEIMER'S

The incidences of premature Alzheimer's are becoming more frequent, and unfortunately, people are deteriorating to the point of being non-functional.

CASE STUDY

Recently, I saw a sixty-nine-year-old patient who flew F-16 fighter missions in Vietnam. After the war, he was a pilot for Delta Airlines for twenty-five years and supervised pilot training for seven years after he retired. His wife brought him in to the clinic, frustrated and concerned. His physical appearance was good; trim and healthy. He was a vibrant, highly capable man, but for some reason his memory and cognitive ability had vastly deteriorated. When I talked to him, he understood me for the most part, but when I asked him to talk, he couldn't find any words. He had been to many neurologists—his brain MRI and all related tests were normal, so the doctors diagnosed him with premature Alzheimer's.

I asked him to get up, walk over to a table, and sit down. He followed my instructions, but when I asked, "How are you feeling?" He couldn't respond. I could tell he was looking for words—he just couldn't find them. Through physical exam and lab testing, I discovered many issues with his health—he had significant nutritional deficiencies. He had low blood amino acids, vitamin D, magnesium, and zinc; bad gut bacteria and parasites; and low levels of the neurotransmitters dopamine, GABA, and serotonin. He also tested positive for Lyme disease. We took one look at all of these abnormalities, and we could see why the most important organ in his body—his brain—was not functioning well. If the brain is not receiving adequate nutrition, it just won't work, because the brain has high energy requirements, using about 20 percent of all the energy in the body. Since essential amino acids are the building blocks of all enzymes and neurotransmitters, they must be in abundant supply at all times to maintain brain health. These cases are very tragic, but with proper nutritional support, including essential amino acids, the elderly can improve their brain function for a better quality of life.

CASE STUDY

In another case related to what was thought to be Alzheimer's, a four-star World War II general brought his ninety-three-year-old wife to see me. They had been married for seventy-two years, but she no longer recognized him; she wouldn't let him sleep in the same bed with her. She had been to several neurologists, yet none of them had been able to help.

Through testing we discovered that she was very protein malnourished, lead-toxic, and saddled with other issues. Perfect Amino was part of her therapy, and after about six months of treatment she improved to the point where she knew everyone's name in the clinic, could count to one hundred, and most importantly, recognized her husband! One day, she brought in a scrapbook from her childhood, identified every person, and told me the story behind every picture. It was obvious that Perfect Amino played a big role in repairing her brain.

The success of her treatment sparked curiosity and motivation in her ninety-two-year-old husband. He loved to play golf, but could no longer see the ball due to macular degeneration. We created a similar nutrition program for him using Perfect Amino; after three months, he scored a documented two-line improvement on the eye chart. He could see the golf ball again and went out to beat his seventy-two-year-old son in a game!

THE CONNECTION TO REDUCED MUSCLE MASS AND WEAKENED IMMUNE SYSTEMS

It's impossible to prevent all age-related breakdowns, but they can definitely be slowed down and whole-body performance can improve. When we contrast MRI images of a person's arm muscles at age twenty and fifty, we can see that the average person loses about thirty percent of their lean body weight throughout those years. Normally, this is considered a byproduct of aging, but studies completed at USC show that the cells of an older person can make protein just as well as those of a twenty-year-old—the real problem is that their dietary habits and poor GI function don't supply their bodies with the nutrients they need to maintain lean body mass.

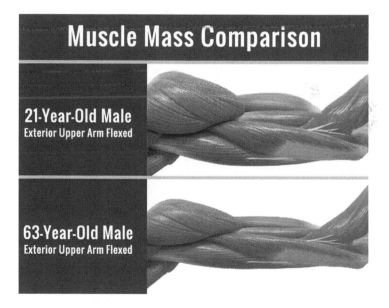

Muscle Mass Comparison

21-Year-Old Male
Exterior Upper Arm Flexed

63-Year-Old Male
Exterior Upper Arm Flexed

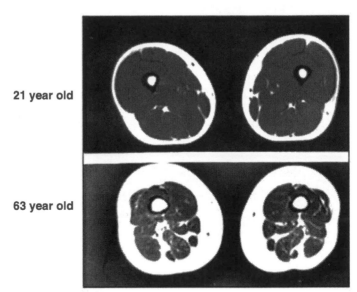

21 year old

63 year old

Age-related changes in muscle mass in thigh cross-sectional area of two people with similar BMI

Another issue with many older people is that they aren't using or stressing their muscles like they used to. For example, when I was forty, there were three hundred men in my age group for Ironman races. Now that I'm seventy, and there are usually only ten or twenty. Most men my age are retired and have the time to commit to training, and I believe many of them would if their bodies weren't broken down. Those who continue to train and maintain their performance are doing the right things physically and nutritionally.

The elderly have also spent a lifetime living with environmental toxins, which is another cause of health issues and systematic breakdown. Their intestinal membranes are thin, and there is a delayed turnover of the inner-lining cells—this makes them more susceptible to diverticulitis and infections. Normal intestinal cell turnover should occur every three or four days, but without enough essential amino acids, vitamins, and minerals, it might happen every seven to ten days—this means that the membranes are not as strong as they should be. The junctions where membranes meet can become unsealed, and bacteria can work their way into the urinary tract or bloodstream. Also, our blood contains immune proteins called *immunoglobulins* that protect us from infection, but if they are low, our ability to resist a virus or bacteria decreases. Amino acids are required to keep your immunoglobulin levels up.

If one can maintain their nutrition throughout the years, they will stay active and mentally competent—nutrition is the most important factor of healthy aging. Essential amino acids are also key, so I make it a habit to never miss a dose. I want to be doing Ironman races well into my eighties and beyond!

CHAPTER NINE

SPECIFIC TO CHILDREN

My practice has a strong interest in the effect of protein on the overall health of autistic children. Many autistic children are sensitive to textures and smells, and most don't like meat, fish, or eggs; they like French fries. They often have a horrible diet, and it's not because their parents don't try their best—the kids simply won't eat it. If they dislike the texture, they won't eat it, and you can't force a two-year-old to eat!

We've found that autistic kids are loaded with environmental toxins. These are often acquired from their mothers in the womb, as it is known that the mother will "detox" into the placenta, and then into the baby. Then, after birth, heavy amounts of substances like mercury, aluminum, and formaldehyde enter their system from vaccinations, which adds to the load. Newborns suck on plastic bottle nipples and pacifiers; chemically-laced, flame retardant parts on their cribs; and GMO laden baby cereals laced with pesticides. When they get older, they crawl around on the floor and in the grass, and they're exposed to more chemicals and pesticides. They don't stand a chance! Children's systems are overwhelmed the moment their lives begin, and if they lack good nutrition, they will exhibit developmental delays and may not be able to adequately detoxify to maintain their health.

Babies need to receive excellent nutrition so they can grow and develop to their full genetic endowment. As you know very well at this point, the main structure of the body is protein, and proteins are made of amino acids. For children who are finicky protein eaters, or autistic children who refuse it, our Perfect AminoXP drink mix in berry or lemon-lime flavor goes down easily, and kids are usually happy to take it. Parents put a half-scoop in a few ounces of water, and the kids drink it down. It tastes good to them, and it's an effective way to get protein and essential amino acids into children who don't eat enough meat or fish to maintain healthy bodies.

THE CONNECTION TO GROWING CHILDREN

Some parents are successful in getting their kids to eat nutritious, balanced meals, and some are not. We know many parents who supplement their kids' diets with Perfect Amino, and just like adults, they have more energy and recover faster after playing sports.

The coaches of a local soccer team and gymnastics team rave about how much better the kids recover when they get enough protein—they are less sore and exhibit better endurance. The benefit continues throughout the higher education years as well: A PAC 10 school's championship program swimming coach has his athletes take Perfect Amino, and he believes it's had a big impact on their performance. In athletics, recovery is the key to consistent performance and adequate protein intake makes that possible.

CASE STUDY

A newborn was born with gastroschisis, a condition in which the skin and muscles don't close over the intestines, and the abdomen is wide open at birth. Doctors gradually stretched his skin over the first few weeks of his life to get the gap to close. They were able to sew the skin shut, but his abdomen was so tight that his intestines couldn't function.

Since the baby couldn't eat, he was given food through an IV called hyperalimentation. This was his sole source of nutrition, and it contained everything he needed to survive. He could take almost no nutrition by mouth for seven or eight months. Kids on hyperalimentation can get hepatitis from the IV proteins, and unfortunately, this child developed the disease. He turned yellow, and the hospital staff couldn't give him the hyperalimentation protein any longer. After seven months, he was still in the hospital and only weighed seven pounds; he hadn't grown at all. His mother checked him out of the hospital on a two-hour pass and brought him in to see me.

We began to give the baby half a gram of Perfect Amino per pound of body weight. His mother mashed up a tablet with a bit of applesauce and water, and the child could easily take it. He began to grow and put on weight within the first two weeks. Since he could now take in protein, his hepatitis cleared, and his gut began to function properly. With only half a tablet of Perfect Amino three times a day, his weight gain increased to the normal rate for infants—he gained a pound or two each week until he caught up to his peers. By age two, he was like any other child in size and development. This is an inspiring, remarkable story and a testament to the power of Perfect Amino.

THE CONNECTION TO PREGNANT WOMEN AND NURSING MOTHERS

An issue with pregnancy today is that women don't spend six months getting themselves into optimal health before getting pregnant. When the mother is unhealthy, the baby becomes a dump site for the toxins in her body. If a mother is toxic, she can take Perfect Amino and consult with a doctor to create a whole-body detox and nutrition program to benefit herself and her baby.

We know healthy moms make healthy babies, and I believe the healthiest babies come from mothers who have taken Perfect Amino during pregnancy and nursing. Breast milk from Perfect Amino mothers is a beautiful, of creamy consistency, and high in nutritive value. Supplementing with Perfect Amino while nursing not only creates wonderful breast milk, but it benefits the mother's health, also. Nursing mothers are often exhausted and may not be eating well, so they deplete their own body protein to feed their child—it's only a matter of time before her bones, organs, and immune system break down.

Pregnant mothers must consider the nutritional needs for two people. They must ensure that their growing fetus receives optimal nutrition to engineer a healthy, perfect body, and they have to keep their own nutrition up in order for that to happen. They also must be healthy enough to nurse for a year or two, without breaking down their own health. For these reasons, attention to essential amino acids prior to, during, and after pregnancy is of the utmost importance.

CHAPTER TEN

FATIGUE, DEPRESSION, AND INSOMNIA

We have many clients—male and female—who have problems with low energy, depression, and insomnia. These add to the list of epidemics in our culture that we didn't see twenty-five years ago. What makes it even more alarming is that we see it in children, too.

There are roughly eight million children taking psych medications for Attention Deficit Disorder (ADD) and Attention Deficit/Hyperactivity Disorder (ADHD). There's no doubt that these children and adults may be symptomatic and unhealthy, but diagnosing anyone with a psychiatric disorder and prescribing mind-altering drugs like Ritalin or Adderal is not the solution. Medications may bring apparent relief, but it's only temporary—these drugs will damage the brain and nervous system in the long run.[15] Many people come into our practice with symptoms of depression, anxiety, and brain fog, and we measure neurotransmitter levels in these cases. These neurotransmitters include serotonin, dopamine, GABA, glutamate, epinephrine, and norepinephrine, and symptomatic patients always have levels that are far below the optimal standards. Even when they have been given prescription psych medications by their doctor, their levels remain low because the drugs do not correct the underlying cause. These medications don't correct the deficiency—they poison the nerves so they are not able to regulate in a normal manner.

For example, the class of drugs called selective serotonin reuptake inhibitors (SSRIs), like Prozac, artificially increase levels of serotonin. Under normal circumstances, when one nerve communicates with another, it shoots a serotonin molecule across a synapse. The molecule then hits the second nerve, and it reacts. The original nerve then uses suction to reel the serotonin back in. SSRIs essentially poison the suction of the first nerve, so it can't reuptake the serotonin—it sits in the synapse and bombards the second nerve cell membrane until it loses sensitivity. The nerve cell membrane is overwhelmed and damaged—the structure changes over time, and it

15   Lavitt, John, "Research Shows Ritalin Causes Long-Term Brain Injury," The Fix, April 14, 2014, https://www.thefix.com/content/research-shows-ritalin-causes-long-term-brain-injury

becomes numb.[16] Subsequently, the symptoms are suppressed, but the underlying problem—which often times is nutritional—is never truly addressed.

These drugs are dangerous because they can randomly affect many nerve cells, and severe side effects have been reported including suicide, mania, and psychotic homicidal behavior. Sometimes psychiatric medications send people over the edge—they become violent and kill someone, or they commit suicide. In fact, it has been documented that many of the mass murderers of the past thirty years had been under psychiatric care, and had SSRIs or other psych drugs in their bloodstreams at the time of their rampages.[17]

We help patients wean off these medications by repairing the inflamed intestines (where 90 percent of serotonin is made) through dietary changes, removal of toxic yeast, bacteria and parasites, and targeted nutrition including essential amino acids to heal the membrane. Once we begin this process, the body begins producing neurotransmitters as it should. We temporarily give them amino acid precursors so the body can make its own serotonin, GABA, or dopamine. In most cases, we measure

16 "Antidepressants—Brain Damage and Chronic Brain Impairments," Toxic Psychiatry, http://www.toxicpsychiatry.com/antidepressant-brain-damage

17 "Antidepressants are a Prescription for Mass Shootings," Citizens Commission on Human Rights, Florida, https://www.cchrflorida.org/antidepressants-are-a-prescription-for-mass-shootings

neurotransmitter levels again six to nine months later, and they have come into normal range. Once those levels are normal, patients can wean off their medication without drastic side effects. This approach is effective because we address the root of the problem; we don't just put up a window dressing in the form of a drug.

18   Netz Y, "Is the Comparison between Exercise and Pharmacologic Treatment of Depression in the Clinical Practice Guideline of the American College of Physicians Evidence-Based?" PubMed Central, May 15, 2017, https://www.ncbi.nlm.nih.gov/pmc/articles/PMC5430071/

19   Reese, Hope, "The Real Problems with Psychiatry," the atlantic.com, May 2, 2013, https://www.theatlantic.com/health/archive/2013/05/the-real-problems-with-psychiatry/275371/

20   Amen, Daniel G; Trujillo, Manuel; Newberg, Andrew; Willeumier, Kristen; Tarzwell, Robert; Wu, Joseph C; Chaitin, Barry, "Brain SPECT Imaging in Complex Psychiatric Cases: An Evidence-Based, Underutilized Tool," National Center for Biotechnology Information, July 28, 2011, https://www.ncbi.nlm.nih.gov/pmc/articles/PMC3149839

PSYCHIATRIC "DIAGNOSES"

Psychiatry is an industry that has no objective proof of its diagnoses. Psychiatrists don't conduct lab tests to confirm their findings, they don't measure neurotransmitter levels, and they don't image the brain to look for structural changes that may be affecting its function. Due to the subjective nature of this industry, three different psychiatrists can have three different "diagnoses" for one patient.

I believe that psychiatry perpetrates fraud on innocent human beings. Clinical studies have proven that exercise is as effective as any drug for treating depression,[18] yet psychiatrists swear by their Bible of "diseases," *The Diagnostic and Statistical Manual* (DSM). This is an extensive list of psychiatric diagnoses with diagnostic codes, so that insurance companies can be billed properly. The tome is nine hundred-forty-three pages long and lists three hundred-seventy-four mental "disorders." This manual is the engine that drives a $330 billion industry, and it's used to enforce psychiatric drugging, seize your children, and even take away your most precious freedoms. Psychiatrists literally sit in a room and make up diagnoses of mental conditions. Then they vote on them, and just like that, we have a new, codeable "mental" disease.[19] Some of these made up diseases include math anxiety disorder, narcissistic personality disorder, and trichotillomania disorder (twisting your hair until it falls out).

I wish I was joking about all of this but, sadly, I am not. I advise you to beware, because psychiatry can hurt you. They have abandoned the old practice of lending a sympathetic ear to the grieved or distressed, and traded it for drugs and electroshock therapy—it turns people into zombies, and that is not the type of help or care that we need.

Now, there are doctors outside the circle of traditional psychiatry who will do objective testing on the brain. One such method is a single-photon emission computerized tomography (SPECT) scan, which can view circulation patterns of the brain. A SPECT scan allows doctors to see old trauma that may have been too minor to be recognized at the time of an injury, and can also indicate the presence of environmental mold, toxins, and even Lyme disease.[20] This practice can actually lead to a true revelation of the patient's condition, so that the underlying problem can be resolved.

CASE STUDY

A sixteen-year-old male, Joseph, came to our clinic from out of state with serious anxiety and depression. This disease had changed his whole outlook on life—he was sullen during his first visit, and he wouldn't look at me or speak to me. He also had a "gothic" look: his hair was dyed black, he wore all black clothing, and had huge earrings and other heavy chains on his arms, neck, and wrists. He told me that "he could not stand to be in his own skin." He had been given all varieties of psych drugs which only made him feel worse. The radiologist gave us a heads up that he could have Lyme disease, and his SPECT scan confirmed his theory to be true. We also discovered that his intestine was growing toxic bacteria, yeast and two parasites; his serum essential amino acid levels were low; he tested positive for several infections in addition to Lyme disease; and he had very low levels of serotonin, which is associated with depression; and GABA, which is related to anxiety.

With comprehensive approaches including natural medicine to correct each of these problems, within four months, Joseph's depression and anxiety were no longer a problem. He washed the dye out of his hair and took off the gothic clothes and jewelry. During his exit interview he said, "I was not myself. I didn't know what was wrong, and I was sure no one could ever help me. But now I feel like I'm back, and I am looking forward to life—my first goal is to get my driver's license. I am so grateful that my mom dragged me here so I could get help."

AMINO ACIDS AND THE CONNECTION TO THE NERVOUS SYSTEM

The vast majority of molecules in the brain and nervous system are made from amino acids. Growth hormone from the pituitary gland, dopamine from the *substantia nigra* area of the brain, and the aforementioned neurotransmitters, serotonin, GABA, epinephrine, norepinephrine, and glutamate are all amino acid based. If there are amino acid deficiencies in the brain, as well as cofactor deficiencies of Vitamin B6 and magnesium, then there can't be adequate production of these protein molecules. If you add in mold, environmental toxins, or infections such as Lyme, mycoplasma, and other bugs, the brain can't operate normally—people can suffer from all sorts of maladies like anxiety and depression, balance issues and vertigo, and poor sleep. Contrary to popular belief, most of these conditions are medical or nutritional—they are not psychological. That is why psychiatry has such dismal success: it assumes that everyone has a drug deficiency and does not take into account external emotional factors or physical illnesses. It offers one misguided solution, rather than addressing what is truly wrong.

It's important to understand that when people don't "feel right," their neurotransmitters are out of whack, and it's most likely because their intestinal flora is out of balance, and they are deficient in key nutrients like essential amino acids. Instead of seeing a psychiatrist, they should get help from a nutritional practitioner who is knowledgeable in such matters. It's true that many issues and situations in life feel like a downward spiral, but taking a drug to numb the symptoms is not the solution—you must find and treat the root cause of the problem. A combination of correct nutritional therapy and effective practical help can alleviate the condition or challenge that has put one into an emotional or spiritual upheaval.

WOMEN AND DEPRESSION

I observed a group of women some years ago who suffered from a triad of symptoms: depression, fatigue, and sleeplessness. Each of them had been on medication long term to block the production of stomach acid, like Nexium, Tagamet, Pepcid, Zantac, or others. I discovered that each woman's blood level of the essential amino acid, tryptophan, was very low.

The usual medical approach to treat women who have this triad of fatigue, insomnia, and depression is to give them prescriptions for Ambien, Trazadone, or Xanax for sleep; Prozac or another SSRI for the depression; and Adderall or another amphetamine for fatigue. And of course, they are to continue taking the acid blocker that caused their problems in the first place.

---

21 Watanabe, J. H., McInnis, T., & Hirsch, J. D. (2018). Cost of Prescription Drug-Related Morbidity and Mortality. Annals of Pharmacotherapy, 52(9), 829–837. doi:10.1177/1060028018765159

22 Persaud, Raj; Bruggen, Peter, "Why Do Patients Stop Dying When Doctors Go on Strike?" psychologytoday.com, October 17, 2015, https://www.psychologytoday.com/us/blog/slightly-blighty/201510/why-do-patients-stop-dying-when-doctors-go-strike

THE TRAGEDY OF IATROGENIC ILLNESS

Ever wonder why the third leading cause of death in the U.S. is iatrogenic (doctor caused) illness? If you multiply the case examples in this book by the millions of therapies that cause a problem, and then overlay that with more drugs to handle the therapy-induced problems, the end result is two hundred-twenty-five to four hundred forty thousand iatrogenic deaths per year. This is evidence that medical practices are in need of a very thorough overhaul. These deaths are a tragedy of immense proportions, hiding behind the veil of "the best medicine in the world."

The University of San Diego reports expenses resulting from medication failures and medication-related issues totaling $495 to $672 billion per year. In addition to this unnecessary expense, there are also an estimated 275,689 deaths per year,[21] and *Psychology Today* reports that when doctors go on strike, patient death rates can actually *decrease!*[22]

To further put this into perspective, imagine that these hundreds of thousands of deaths were the result of something else, like plane crashes. If three large aircrafts carrying two hundred-twenty-five people each crashed on a daily basis all year long, you probably wouldn't be so quick to board an airplane. The risk is just as great when taking unnecessary prescription medications or submitting to questionable surgeries, yet most people don't hesitate to put drugs in their bodies or go under the knife.

So, what exactly was going on with these women? Since you're this far into the book, I'm sure you've got the sequence figured out:

1. Stomach acid-blocking medications blocked the digestion of dietary proteins and the absorption of minerals, like magnesium.
2. Dietary proteins are the source of tryptophan, but since digestion was compromised, tryptophan and other amino acids were not well absorbed. Therefore, their blood levels of tryptophan were low, leading to low levels in the cells.
3. Magnesium and vitamin B6 are needed to make tryptophan into proteins, but they also require stomach acid. Blocking the acid further compromised protein synthesis.
4. Tryptophan is the parent molecule for niacin. Inadequate tryptophan means inadequate niacin, so the cells couldn't make energy. This led to the women having fatigue.
5. Tryptophan is also the parent molecule for melatonin. Since there was inadequate melatonin in their bodies, they couldn't sleep well.
6. Tryptophan is also the parent molecule for serotonin. Low serotonin meant that the ladies were apt to suffer from depression and other mood problems.

These women were fatigued, sleepless, and depressed due to the long-term use of drugs that blocked stomach acid. This was not entirely their own doing—their doctors had dutifully renewed their prescriptions despite the warning in the Physician's Desk Reference that these drugs were for short term use only. This observation led to a very simple solution: We gave them stomach acid supplements containing pancreatic enzymes so they could digest proteins, weaned them off their acid blockers, and gave them essential amino acids with extra tryptophan, B6, B complex, and magnesium. Their fatigue, depression, and sleeplessness all resolved within a few months time. Good detective work combined with nutritional medicine can solve health problems—it's modern medicine at its best!

CHAPTER ELEVEN

WEIGHT-RELATED ISSUES

Many patients will resort to severe calorie restriction in an attempt to lose weight. A popular diet that cycles through the overweight community every ten years or so is called the Human Chorionic Gonadotropin (HCG) diet, which only allows five hundred calories per day for three to six weeks. The hormone HCG is also injected during this time, because it resets the pituitary gland—the person will lose their food cravings and selectively burn fat.

Researchers have found that for every four pounds that a person loses on such a diet, one pound of that is lean body tissue. If someone loses thirty pounds, it means they are losing a significant amount of bone, muscle, and organ tissue. The person may be thinner, but their body composition will be poor. To make matters worse, as soon as the person stops restricting calories, they're likely to return to their old eating habits and gain the weight back within a year—and most of it will be fat without lean body mass. With the loss of lean body mass, their body burns fewer calories, and the weight will pile on again in no time. (And this is true over 90 percent of the time, no matter which diet people attempt.)

However, we have found that if our patients take Perfect Amino while following a calorie-restricted diet, they will get enough protein (with almost no calories), so they are able to maintain lean body mass. To give an example, we tracked the body composition of more than three hundred people who were on HCG diets for twenty-one days. The average male lost fifteen to twenty pounds, and the average female lost twelve to fifteen pounds. The patients who were given Perfect Amino maintained their lean body mass during these periods of rapid weight loss, so their overall outcome was much better—Perfect Amino helps prevent the breakdown of their bodies and maintain overall health.

Another published study examined a group of people who ate only fruits and vegetables that amounted to two thousand calories per day, along with essential amino acids in Perfect Amino as their sole protein source. They took ten grams (ten tablets) of the essential amino acids daily. After four weeks, each person had lost an average of three pounds per week, and they had maintained their lean body mass—their skin even retained its elasticity.[23]

At the time of this writing, there is a great interest in the benefits of fasting for improving health and reducing the risk of cancer. People are advised to go twenty-four hours, up to even a week, just drinking water or non-caloric tea. In my own experience, adding essential amino acids as a part of a fast makes the process go much better. The body needs amino acids while fasting to support liver detoxification—it needs to get rid of the accumulated toxic matter that is being released from the cells. Also, during a fast, the body attempts to rebuild its internal structure, and adequate amino acid intake facilitates this process. Patients find that the fast goes easier when they supplement with amino acids, and they spare their lean body mass—they don't end up weak and depleted.

Amino acids are the core of life; they are necessary to keep the body moving along, to heal, and to recover. It doesn't matter if you're trying to build muscle, recover from an operation or infection, or just maintain your health against the onslaughts of daily life—amino acids are essential and should never be neglected.

---

23   Lucà-Moretti M; Grandi A; Lucà E; Muratori G; Nofroni MG; Mucci MP; Gambetta P; Stimolo R; Drago P; Giudice G; Tamburlin N; "Master Amino acid Pattern as substitute for dietary proteins during a weight-loss diet to achieve the body's nitrogen balance equilibrium with essentially no calories." National Center for Biotechnology Information, September 2003, https://www.ncbi.nlm.nih.gov/pubmed/14964348

CHAPTER TWELVE

PROTEINS AND THE KIDNEY AND LIVER

Several million people in the U.S. have serious issues with their kidneys or liver. Sometimes, these issues occur post infection—the person may have had hepatitis B or C and the chronic inflammation damaged the liver. Or, the person took a medication that caused liver or kidney damage. Other times, the damage is caused by an auto-immune condition. Whatever the cause, if either (or both) of these organs aren't functioning well, the body can become toxic.

As we discussed previously, proteins have a molecule of nitrogen as part of their structure, whereas carbs and fats do not. When a protein is broken down, nitrogen is released. In this form, it's toxic for the body, so it's turned into urea by the liver, and then excreted by the kidneys. Any problem or dysfunction with either of these two organs can cause the nitrogen to build up and poison the body. This is known as *uremia*.

If you recall from our previous discussion, liver packages the nitrogen into urea—so if the liver is not working, the nitrogen builds up. In cases of kidney failure, there may be no effective urine output and the level of *blood urea nitrogen* can increase, making them very sick. They might even have to go on dialysis to remove the urea from their body. The common, routine blood test BUN is used to measure levels of blood urea nitrogen. If the level of blood urea nitrogen increases, this indicates that the kidneys may be damaged. We've seen urea levels in sick people increase from ten to twenty, up to fifty and one hundred, with the higher numbers indicating renal failure. This toxic build-up can also cause heart failure, loss of consciousness, seizures, or even death.

For these reasons, people with serious liver and kidney disease are often put on low-protein diets to reduce the amount of nitrogen entering their bodies. These diets include a lot of vegetables and starches, but high-protein foods like meats, fish, eggs, dairy, and beans are limited. This is problematic because we need protein to keep our immune system and body tissues at full strength. People on low protein diets can become anemic (low levels of blood), have muscle loss that leads to weakness, skin breakdown, osteoporosis, lowered immune proteins, and heart failure. Not only that, but if patients are on dialysis, the mechanical trauma to their blood cells causes them to break, and it further worsens anemia—without enough protein, people can waste away or get serious infections.

The perfect solution for protein-restricted kidney and liver patients is for them to get their daily protein in the form of Perfect Amino. This complete protein produces less than 1 percent nitrogen waste, so it can supplement their diets and improve their overall nutrition. Very few nephrologists, hepatologists, or liver specialists know about this product, so if you are a kidney or liver patient, you should coordinate this with your personal physician.

If every person on dialysis took Perfect Amino, they could reduce their treatment frequency by 30 percent. It would save tens of millions of dollars every year, while enhancing their quality of life.

THE CONNECTION TO CANCERS

We treat cancer patients in my practice, and due to the physical impact of radiation or chemotherapy treatments, many of them have no appetite. They're sick, nauseous, and often hit with diarrhea. Without adequate nutrition, they can't take in enough protein—their bodies slowly deteriorate and their susceptibility to infection sky-rockets. They're hit with a double whammy of sickness and malnourishment.

An indicator of their future prognosis is often found in their level of total serum protein. This can be measured through routine testing as part of a complete metabolic panel. When the total drops below normal—about five and a half—that tells us that a cancer patient won't live much longer, unless we can get them enough digestible and absorbable protein to increase their level.

We've found that if we give our cancer patients high doses of Perfect Amino, we can often recover their total serum protein, improve their lean body mass, and improve anemia. They can take ten grams of the tablets or powdered preparation three times a day, and this prevents their bodies from breaking down. It makes a big difference in their prognosis and recovery, and there's no downside—we're not giving them an artificial product or sugary food.

MORE ON THE PROTEIN PROBLEM AND LEAKY GUT

Due to the amount of pesticides in foods, the hormones and antibiotics fed to the animals we eat, and ubiquitous prescriptions of drugs, many people today suffer from leaky gut. Even something seemingly harmless—like aspirin—can cause problems. A common recommendation is to take aspirin every day to prevent a heart attack. However, even in small doses, aspirin and other pharmaceutical drugs can cause injury to the stomach and small intestine, bleeding of the intestinal lining, and a leaky gut.

The gut requires adequate amounts of essential amino acids to regenerate itself every few days. If they are lacking in the body, then the gut membrane can become more permeable, creating an increased susceptibility to "leak" fragments from proteins and microorganisms into the bloodstream from the intestines. Some people even contract infections *from their own intestines*, which can lead to a serious blood infection, resulting in sepsis or meningitis.

High doses of essential amino acids are required to keep the intestinal membrane intact. Since Perfect Amino is predigested, doesn't require enzymes, and contains no residue or fiber, the body readily absorbs it for use in making protein. They are simply pure, pharmaceutical grade amino acids in L-form, the form that is used by the body. Once it hits the small intestines, there's nothing left to be digested, handled, or defecated.

Nearly all of today's autoimmune diseases such as lupus, rheumatoid arthritis, and multiple sclerosis stem from leaky intestines, and if those are healed, people can regain health. However, most medical professionals don't pay much attention to this. We know that the traditional dietician still counts protein grams and thinks they are all the same, when in fact, they are not—they don't all function and repair in the same way. Refer to chapter 1 for more on net amino acid utilization.

SYMPTOMS AND IDENTIFICATION OF A LEAKY GUT

In many cases, people have lived with symptoms of leaky gut for so long that they think it's normal. Bloating, gas or heartburn, gastroesophageal reflux disease (GERD), constipation or the opposite, and bad breath are all just a part of life; they aren't viewed as maladies that have a specific cause.

Not long ago, a nurse came to my office in a wheelchair. She had MS and was unable to walk. I asked her about her bowel habits because nearly 100 percent of people with a neurological illness have chronic constipation. If you're not moving out a stool mass at least once a day, guess what? It goes back in, and you'll suffer from autointoxication because the waste is going the wrong way. Virtually everyone I see with Parkinson's, dementia, Alzheimer's, ALS, or MS is constipated. Rarely do people with these conditions have a happy intestine, flat stomach, and full evacuation every day.

This nurse was in her 40s, and when I asked about her bowel habits she said, "It's normal. I have a bowel movement at least every couple of weeks. It's been like that for a long time." She didn't realize she had been constipated since childhood! Children get cramps with constipation and are unable to defecate, but after a while the intestines stop fighting it; the body stops complaining. Children decide early on "that's just how I am," and they carry that non-solution into adulthood. Because of that, this nurse thought every couple of weeks was normal.

Of course, we know that is *not* normal. Every patient I've seen with chronic illness had leaky intestines—they were colonized with parasites, fungus, and unhealthy bacteria. Once an intestine leaks, it absorbs substances that can lead to allergies, sinus problems, and recurrent tonsillitis. People with this condition end up on antibiotics because they get infections. Antibiotics kill good bacteria, so the person is left with only the bad—this causes local inflammation and leaks bio toxins into the body, further poisoning it. It becomes a vicious cycle.

MEASURING CRP AND MICROBIOMES

We screen all patients for artery disease with a high-sensitivity test that measures their C-reactive protein (CRP). This is a protein that increases when inflammation is present in the blood or its vessels. Three is considered average, but the ideal level is below one. Sadly, I've seen levels as high as thirty. Someone with an elevated CRP is at a higher risk of developing clots in their heart, brain, or other arteries, and even cancer.

The cause of an elevated CRP is almost always one of two things: a chronically infected tooth (within the root canal), or gums (gingivitis, deep pockets), or a chronic intestinal infection. With the former, bacteria enter the bloodstream through pockets in the gums or infected teeth. With a chronic intestinal infection, we can conduct a stool test and grow out the bacteria to analyze its profile. Typically, we find that they have yeasts and/or two to four high-level toxic bugs like *Pseudomonas*, *Kiebsiella*, and *Proteus*. These infectious bacteria cause local inflammation/infection in the gut, and they produce bio toxic waste that is absorbed across the intestinal membrane, poisoning other cells in a remote location. They are true enemies living within us.

We can test the bio toxin levels produced by these bacteria or yeasts in a urine specimen from the patient. Since the toxins cross the intestinal membrane and enter the bloodstream, they are eventually filtered out by the kidney and show up in the urine. These bio toxins may have entered the inner lining of the arteries along the way, causing inflammation and then plaque formation. Or, they may have entered the brain and poisoned neu-

HEALTHY GUT, HEALTHY BODY

Hippocrates said it best in 400 B.C: "Disease begins in the colon." The first area of concern when someone has a chronic condition of any kind is the intestine—they knew it back then, and yet modern gastroenterologists don't look at the microbiome (intestinal flora) as the key to health. For example, if you have GERD, you will be scoped, and if they find H. Pylori, you're instructed to take three different antibiotics for that infection. Your intestine will be out of sorts for months! With colitis, you're given antibiotics or steroids without a care for actually healing the intestine. Someone given a course of antibiotics has a better than 20 percent chance of feeling depressed or anxious due to the disturbance of the microbiome caused by the antibiotic. There is no health without intestinal health.

rons causing brain fog, depression, or sleep problems. When we are able to clear out these harmful organisms, the patient feels better, and the toxins produced by the bacteria go away.

To maintain good health, we must nurture our bodies by eating the proper food and staying away from medicines, except in extreme emergency situations. To that end, we work with patients over three-to-six-month periods to rehabilitate their microbiome so they have a healthy, non-leaking gut, and are free from bloating, gas, constipation, and heartburn—we want those ailments to be a thing of the past. Following treatment, many people remark, "I don't have intestinal symptoms anymore, and my gut feels really good. I never thought the problem would be solved." Restoring the gut is the first step toward restoring a person's health, and it's always my highest priority when treating any sick patient.

THE GUT-BRAIN

We've known for a long time that you cannot have a healthy brain without a healthy intestine. We find a diseased gut in all patients with neurological disease. The typical neurologist does not have any treatments that will reverse Alzheimer's or Parkinson's disease or improve the condition by reversing the cause. You will not find them considering any treatment besides prescribing drugs to suppress Parkinson's tremors or sedatives to calm the Alzheimer's patient. Drugs for Parkinson's can be helpful for a while, but they don't address the root cause or reverse the disease. People get worse over time, and then they develop other issues—it can get to the point where they lose motor control of their bodies. I've had experience with many of these patients, and if they're not too far gone, the processes and treatments we recommend can actually reverse or at the very least, stabilize their disease. Many of them regain normal function and their symptoms visibly improve. We've seen that the body can heal if given the correct treatments and nutrition.

THE BODY KNOWS WHAT TO DO

The body has ways to protect itself from noxious elements that can be harmful. The body has major external barriers in place, (the skin); and internal barriers (the lining of the nose and mouth), the gastrointestinal tract, the pulmonary (lung) system and the blood-brain barrier, which all help to prevent toxic substances from entering our organs. The one thing that these barriers have in common is that they are all made of protein and phospholipids (structural fats). If there is an inadequate amount of essential amino acids in the body, barrier tissues can get leaky, and the organs are not well protected. Perfect Amino helps to maintain these protective barriers and keep us functional and strong.

CONCLUSION

THE PERFECT PROTEIN

The key takeaway from this book is that you need to eat organic foods and clean sources of healthy protein. I say the following as a doctor and a former vegetarian: vegans and vegetarians who don't supplement their diets with amino acids are very likely to experience a decline in health—there just isn't enough protein in fruits and vegetables to maintain cellular health. If you've been a vegetarian for more than six to twelve months, it is very likely that your level of serum essential amino acids is low, which is the prelude to your body moving into a state of breakdown.

Historically, there have been no long-term vegan or vegetarian populations on Earth, with the exception of small pockets of people here and there—the most plentiful source of good nutrition has always been animal foods. We've had millions of years of exposure to animal proteins and much less time with vegetable proteins as a primary source. I believe that the Paleo diet is good, and most would do well with it, because even though food production practices have changed, our bodies have not. I find that 80 percent of my patients feel healthier just by following an organic Paleo Diet. Again, it's vitally important to have *clean* sources of protein, ideally from animals that were free to roam around, eat their natural foods, were not given hormones and antibiotics, and weren't fed synthetic or GMO foods.

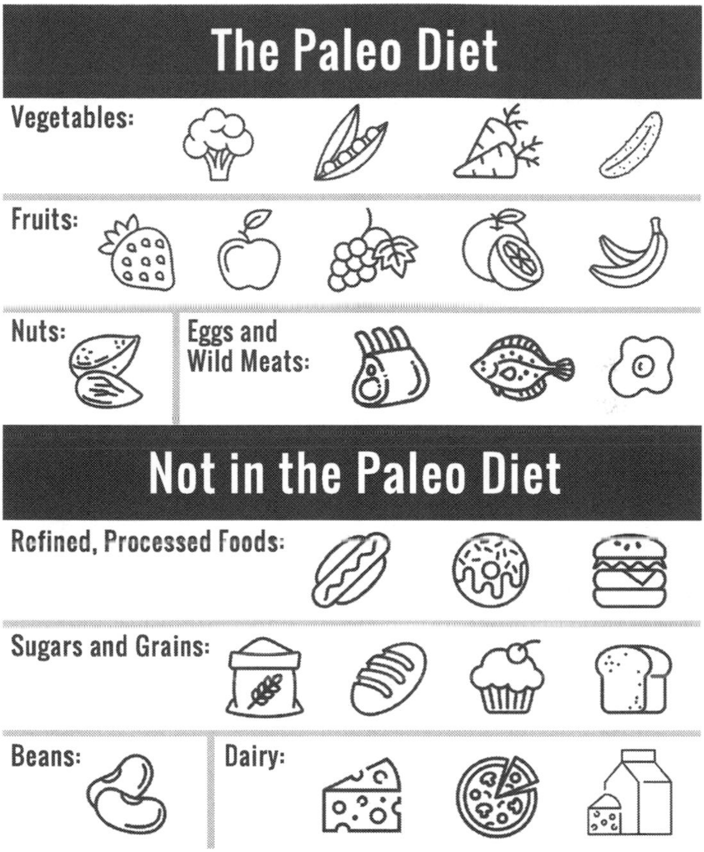

The Paleo Diet

Vegetables:

Fruits:

Nuts: **Eggs and Wild Meats:**

Not in the Paleo Diet

Refined, Processed Foods:

Sugars and Grains:

Beans: **Dairy:**

If you are a vegetarian or vegan for spiritual reasons, or that's just what you've been called to do, more power to you. Just make sure that you are taking care of your complete nutritional needs. If you're on a high-vegetable starch diet, you have to be aware of your intake of essential Omega-3 fats, iron, and B-12. If you're a vegetarian or a vegan, you should take ten tablets of Perfect Amino (or the equivalent) at least once a day to ensure that your protein nutrition is adequate.

IT'S YOUR CHOICE

As important as they are, proteins aren't the only food we need—we need essential fats and oils as well. Animal proteins are good sources for these, especially if we eat ones that were raised in their natural state. They are also a good source of vitamins and minerals. However, in today's world with our depleted soil, most people still don't get the nutrients that they need, so supplementation is required to keep our bodies healthy and strong enough to battle our toxic environment.

The following is my typical dietary recommendation for patients who need to get healthy: "For six weeks, dairy, grains, legumes, and bean products are off limits. No nightshade vegetables like eggplants, peppers, and white potatoes. You will eat meat, fish, eggs, fruits, vegetables, nuts and seeds." The common remark following the diet is: "It took me a week or two to get used to this. I had a bunch of cravings at first, but now I feel better. I have a bowel movement once or twice every day, I've lost eight pounds, my brain feels good, and I sleep better." I usually give patients vitamins and minerals along with some Perfect Amino while they are on this diet, but it's a relatively low-level approach—it can make a difference and promote healing in a person who has been chronically ill.

Food choices are probably the most significant factor in health—they can nurture or kill you, so you have a choice to make: will you slowly kill yourself because you want to eat something that tastes good, or will you find other foods to enjoy that won't harm your body?

THE PERFECT SOLUTION

When most of my patients first come to see me, I find that they have a subclinical protein deficiency. It may not be that they're not eating enough protein—it could be that they're not digesting it well, or they're not absorbing it sufficiently. When they add Perfect Amino as a supplement, it helps them avoid the issues we discussed in this book, or it helps them to begin the process of repair if they have a chronic condition. Most people tolerate the supplement very well—I've given it to tens of thousands of patients, and very, very, few people are allergic or sensitive to it. What's more, it has virtually no calories, it's pre-digested, enzymes are not required, and it's almost completely utilized—it doesn't produce nitrogen waste. If you are concerned about purity, the product is completely vegan and pure, with nothing artificial added. It functions as a supplement for both active and normal lifestyles, and it helps with detoxification. It keeps you nourished, and your skin, hair, nails, brain, and neurotransmitters will be in good shape. It keeps your body in an optimum state, which is where you want to be!

FINAL THOUGHTS

In the final analysis, living a life in good health is mostly a matter of choice. One can choose to eat well, exercise, get enough sleep and sunshine, and take nutritional supplements. One also has a choice as to who they associate with, and we are either nurtured by or emotionally and spiritually harmed by our associations.

We also can't live our lives as the "effect" of everyone and everything. We must take responsibility for our choices and the way we live. If we don't take control, our beliefs will be blown every which way, and we will point to everything else as being the cause for our condition. Even if you do nothing at all, that is still is a choice—you always choose, whether or not you think you do.

Recently, a patient told me, "You tell me to do the opposite of everything I want to do. I like to smoke, eat sugary foods, and drink a lot. And I don't like to exercise." I told him that it was his decision to choose those things. There is no free lunch, and causes have effects. Heart attacks, cirrhosis, lung cancer, COPD, diabetes, and premature Alzheimer's are all effects—they are the price that we pay when we create the causes.

To truly be healthy in today's environment does take some work. Finding good food, non- toxic health and dental care, clean water, and a toxin-free work environment may not be easy, and all can be expensive, but you make the choice—you vote with your wallet and with what you put in your mouth.

HEALTH FOR LIFE

When I was in college, a visiting yogi professor came to lecture us. He said something that I will never forget: "The first twenty years of your life, you can do anything you want. The next twenty, you can coast on grace. The last twenty, your body will take you to hell." He said that in 1978, and unfortunately, it is no longer true.

Gone are those "first twenty years." The incidence of diabetes, obesity, autism, and cancer in children in the first ten years of life is skyrocketing. These are *lifestyle* diseases. Our toxic food, environment, and medical and dental care are the causes of these problems. We have to wake up. The planet and human survival are in a dangerous state. To survive, one must go against the grain (no pun intended) and create healthy habits as though one's life depends on them, because it does. One's habits rules one's life, and one must make good health a habit. The gift of health is one that only *you* can give to yourself—no one else can.

Human biology has strict rules, and violating them can put you in a condition of pain and suffering and possibly premature death. No doctor can save you from yourself. Accidents happen, but I am not talking about those—your keys to health are your daily food and supplements, exercise, sleep, sunshine, and fellowship with like-minded people. Work hard for the betterment of the world around you, and most importantly, nurture yourself as a spiritual being. If you will do those things, you can have health and so thrive; you'll create a life of meaning and purpose, so when your life is near its end, you can look back and say, "I had my time here. I lived and enjoyed, and many were glad that I did."

And for you my friend, I wish that.

Yours in Health,

DM

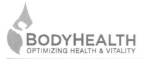

PerfectAmino Uptake and Bioavailability, Plasma Test and Lab Results

Abstract

This study examines the effect of PerfectAmino on the plasma amino acid levels in 5 patients at an Integrative Medical Clinic in Clearwater, FL. Fasting levels of essential serum amino acids and glucose were taken, and then 10 grams of PerfectAmino were fed with repeat serum levels of amino acids and glucose taken at an average of 41 minutes and 103 minutes afterward. The data showed that in every case blood levels of essential amino acids increased significantly from fasting levels with no increase in glucose levels. Additionally, levels of conditionally essential amino acids, (Arginine and Histidine), had increases as well, demonstrating that with PerfectAmino both conditionally essential amino acids can be produced by the body when PerfectAmino is fed. We conclude that PerfectAmino in both tablet and powder from are well absorbed after oral feeding and have no significant effect on blood glucose levels.

Introduction

The goal was to determine A) whether or not the amino acids in the PerfectAmino were absorbable into the bloodstream within the purported short time period with both the tablet and powdered form, B) if the patient's glucose levels were impacted, which would thereby adversely affect those with diabetes or on ketogenic diets and C) does this blend of essential amino acids give the body what it needs to produce the other two so called "conditionally essential" amino acids Arginine and Histidine.

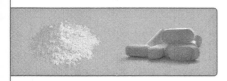

Case Presentation

The question of the utilization and assimilation of PerfectAmino was taken up with this study. Do the

tablets break down in the stomach and upper GI tract and assimilate into the bloodstream quickly? Or do they stay solid and pass through into the lower intestinal tract? Does the powdered form assimilate faster? Can these amino acid blood levels be sustained allowing for the amino acids to be utilized for protein synthesis? Additionally, is the body able to produce the other two essential amino acids, without consuming them directly? And lastly, is there any impact on glucose levels?

Starting on January 9, 2019, 5 patients (3 female and 2 male) arrived for the study in a fasting state and their blood was drawn for baseline levels of serum amino acids and blood glucose. They then consumed 10 tablets of PerfectAmino with a glass of water.

Key Stats

Average Increases:

- 41 minute essential amino acid increase 114%
- 103 minute essential amino acid increase 71%

Glucose levels:

- 41 minute glucose increase 1.5%
- 103 minute glucose increase -1%

Average age of participants: 33 years old
Over base figures

After an average of 38 minutes and then 96 minutes, blood was drawn again, to determine serum levels of amino acids and glucose.

Then on January 10th, the same 5 patients had the same fasting blood draw, after which they consumed 2 scoops of PerfectAminoXP powder (equivalent to 10 tablets). Then after averages of 41 and 103 minutes, their blood was drawn again.

Continued fom page 1

The results in both cases showed that the blood levels of essential amino acids increased within the first 41 minutes and were sustained through and beyond the second test, up to 110 minutes later.

In the case of PerfectAminoXP powder, the 41-minute increase of amino acid levels was at an average of 159%. PerfectAmino tablets showed an increase of 69%, showing faster assimilation into the bloodstream of the powder. In the case of the tablets, the sustained increases after 103 minutes were 77%. The powder had a 66% increase in amino acids in the bloodstream after 103 minutes. Both had similar long term effect on the amino levels, with the main difference being that the tablets had slightly more of a time-release effect.

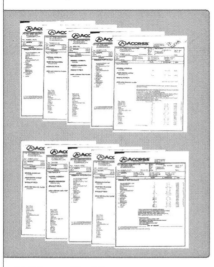

Histidine and Arginine

Both of these are considered conditionally essential amino acids for young children and the elderly and may not naturally be produced by the body. In this study, there were increases of up to 15% in Histidine and 111% in Arginine, despite the fact that the blood draws were in a fasting state and that neither of these amino acids are present in the PerfectAmino tablets or PerfectAminoXP powder.

Glucose

When a protein or amino acids follow the catabolic pathway in the body, they turn in to carbohydrates and sugars and can increase glucose levels, which can have a negative effect on diabetes or those trying to achieve nutritional ketosis. In this case study, there was actually a decrease in the glucose levels, showing definitively that neither PerfectAmino tablets nor PerfectAminoXP powder cause an increase in blood sugar, and thereby can be considered an effective protein source without blood sugar increases or breaking of ketosis, making it "keto friendly."

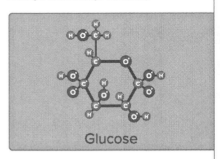

Glucose

Conclusion

In each of these cases, it was evident that the levels of essential amino acids in their blood (including the two that were not present in PerfectAmino) increased significantly and were sustained for the bodies use in protein synthesis. There was evidence that PerfectAmino is as claimed, 99% anabolic and acted as precursors for protein synthesis, and less than 1% of the amino acids were catabolized to produce glucose. While the powder form assimilated more rapidly both it and the tablet form had similar levels of bioavailability. We conclude that PerfectAmino in either powder form or tablet form is the most utilizable amino acid source for protein synthesis and should be a daily supplement for any person wanting optimal body function and health regardless of body age, sex, or activity level.

ABOUT THE AUTHOR

DR. DAVID MINKOFF graduated from the University of Wisconsin Medical School in 1974. He was inducted into the Alpha Omega Alpha Medical Fraternity with high academic honors. He is board certified in pediatrics, completed a fellowship in Infectious Diseases, and served as codirector of the Neonatal Intensive Care Unit at Palomar Medical Center in San Diego, California.

Dr. Minkoff also has extensive post-graduate training in Complementary and Alternative medicine, and cofounded LifeWorks Wellness Center in 1997 with his wife, Sue. In the year 2000, he co-founded BodyHealth, a nutrition company that offers a unique range of dietary supplements to the public and practitioners, including a breakthrough product that the body utilizes over 99 percent for protein synthesis, *PerfectAmino*.

Dr. Minkoff is passionate about fitness, is a forty-two-time IRONMAN finisher, and continues to train on a regular basis. He and his wife reside in Clearwater, Florida.